Child Maltreatment Fatalities in the United States

Emily M. Douglas

Child Maltreatment Fatalities in the United States

Four Decades of Policy, Program, and Professional Responses

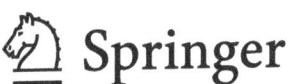 Springer

Emily M. Douglas
Bridgewater State University
Bridgewater, Massachusetts, USA

ISBN 978-94-017-7581-6   ISBN 978-94-017-7583-0 (eBook)
DOI 10.1007/978-94-017-7583-0

Library of Congress Control Number: 2016936372

© Springer Science+Business Media Dordrecht 2017
This work is subject to copyright. All rights are reserved by the Publisher, whether the whole or part of the material is concerned, specifically the rights of translation, reprinting, reuse of illustrations, recitation, broadcasting, reproduction on microfilms or in any other physical way, and transmission or information storage and retrieval, electronic adaptation, computer software, or by similar or dissimilar methodology now known or hereafter developed.
The use of general descriptive names, registered names, trademarks, service marks, etc. in this publication does not imply, even in the absence of a specific statement, that such names are exempt from the relevant protective laws and regulations and therefore free for general use.
The publisher, the authors and the editors are safe to assume that the advice and information in this book are believed to be true and accurate at the date of publication. Neither the publisher nor the authors or the editors give a warranty, express or implied, with respect to the material contained herein or for any errors or omissions that may have been made.

Printed on acid-free paper

This Springer imprint is published by Springer Nature
The registered company is Springer Science+Business Media B.V. Dordrecht

*For Sandra S. Hodge —
my original child welfare mentor and a force
to be reckoned with;
a woman whose priorities are clear,
whose child welfare practice was informed
by evidence,
and who never took her eye off the child.
My professional interests and this book are
because of you.*

Acknowledgments

When I was in graduate school, I studied public policy, family problems, and situations under which children were vulnerable to poor outcomes and sometimes, even harm. It was at this time that I started working for the Maine Child Death & Serious Injury Review Panel (MCDSIRP). This is a multidisciplinary team of professionals with a vested interest in the well being of children in their state, the circumstances that might leave children vulnerable to harm or even death, and the potential gaps in service delivery for such children and their families. I had been working with at-risk children in therapeutic settings such as residential care, specialized school services, and adults in a correctional setting. Thus, I was not completely ignorant to the problems that children and their families can face, but serving on the MCDSIRP was both validating and eye-opening at the same time. My initial work experiences after I finished my undergraduate degree prompted my interest in families and especially the social service systems that support them; I saw these services as fragmented and leaving children in risky situations. The work that I did and the cases that we reviewed on the MCDSIRP confirmed my initial impressions and interactions with the social service sector.

Even more important, as an emerging professional with limited experience, I was surrounded by local giants—professionals from various disciplines who had been working with, investigating, servicing, and treating maltreating families and their children for decades. They made a tremendous impression on me and a lasting mark on my professional aspirations, outlook, and career. I list them here, in alphabetical order.

- Neil Colan, Ed.D., psychologist
- Timothy Doyle, Maine State Police detective
- Michael Ferenc, M.D., medical examiner
- Sandra Hodge, child welfare professional
- Karen Mosher, Ph.D., psychologist
- Lawrence Ricci, M.D., forensic pediatrician

Though from different disciplines, these individuals role-modeled uniform ethical standards that became part of my own professional code of ethics—how to assess for strengths and risks using an approach that is child-centered and safety-centered. They demonstrated for me how a system can support children and their families for optimum physical and emotional well-being, and also taught me to look for gaps in services which can leave a child without a safety net. I have never collectively thanked them for the tremendous impact that they had on my career, my aspirations, and the way that I approach fatal child maltreatment. So, thank you, to each of you—my sincerest gratitude. I must extend a special thank you to Sandra Hodge, who not only planted a seed that led to my interest in child welfare outcomes, but laid a massive oak tree at my feet. More than a decade has passed since she left the child welfare field and she still asks the most important questions of any child welfare practitioner I know. As I noted in my dedication to this book, my professional interests and this book are because of her.

My colleague, Dr. Melinda Gushwa, at Simmons College, has been a constant source of support for me in my work on fatal child maltreatment. With decades of applied social work experience under her belt as a child welfare worker, trainer, medical social worker, clinician, and more, she provides useful insight and role models how practitioners use evidence to inform their approach to working with families. She has walked me through cases, helped me to better understand the systems that support children, listened to my endless concerns about how to balance strengths and risks in child welfare practice, and commiserated with me about children who have needlessly died. It was Melinda who developed the idea of using a "fatality lens," when working with families—a notion that might prevent high risk situations from resulting in death and simultaneously offer more protection for all children. Thank you, Melinda. I look forward to our continued collaborations.

Next, I thank Dr. Dana Mohler-Faria, the recent president of Bridgewater State University in Bridgewater, Massachusetts. He is responsible for the development of the Presidential Fellows Program at this teaching-intensive university, in which each year, one or two faculty are given a year's release from teaching and campus responsibilities to pursue scholarly activities or applied experiences. In the 2010–2011 academic year, Dr. Mohler-Faria, gave me, an untenured faculty member, the opportunity of a lifetime by selecting me as the Presidential Fellow for our institution. This granted me an entire academic year, at full salary, to spend at the Family Research Laboratory at the University of New Hampshire, to focus on the study of fatal child maltreatment. It was during this time that I conducted my research on the intersection of fatal child maltreatment and the child welfare system, and identified the need for a book that would examine the policy, programmatic, and other professional responses to fatal child maltreatment. This opportunity was a pivotal experience in my career and laid the foundation for this book.

I am lucky to have been associated with the Family Research Laboratory and the Crimes Against Children Research Center at the University of New Hampshire since 2002. The weekly research seminars in which one scholar's work in-progress is reviewed in front of a body of peers, has had an important impact on my writing and thinking as a social scientist. Many of the chapters in this book were reviewed by colleagues in this setting; it would be impossible to identify all of the contributions that were made and incorporated into this book. The footprints of their remarks and recommendations are spread through these pages and I am deeply indebted to them. I cannot thank Drs. Murray Straus and David Finkelhor enough; as the "founding fathers" of the study of family violence and child victimization, their sincere interest in my work and ideas have advanced my scholarship on fatal child maltreatment. An extra special thank you to Murray who passed away in May of 2016. He continues to be a daily source of inspiration for me.

There are numerous other people who offered me support in the writing of this book. My research and graduate assistants, Brandy Mohn, Stephen Maloney, and Sarah Cleaver, conducted literature reviews, retrieved articles, compiled databases, edited chapters, obtained copyright permissions, and did all of the "grunt" work that goes with writing a book. Despite these menial tasks, I don't think that I heard a single complaint from any of them. Dr. Jenn Vanderminden, a colleague and one-time officemate at the Family Research Laboratory, listened to me tell countless, ugly stories about deceased children; solved endless statistical quandaries that I could not resolve; shared her chocolate; and, engaged in shared mini therapeutic sessions over the angst that all academics bear. Toni Chance, fellow child welfare professional, has answered many questions about risk factors, child welfare training, and child welfare practice concerning fatal child maltreatment. Her interest, support, and sweet, southern voice have provided reassurance on more than one occasion. Rachel Angerhofer, also another child welfare practitioner, has entertained many questions and asked me questions in turn, which have informed my thinking. She has talked to my students on numerous occasions about the child welfare profession and willingly gave feedback on chapters in this book—all-the-while staying afloat when her own state agency battled several child fatality-related crises. Thank you to Drs. Lars Alberth, Jess Goldberg, Hal Grotevant, Lisa Jones, the now late Staci Perlman, and Wendy Walsh—all stellar colleagues who provided last-minute feedback and advice on my writing and conclusions. Michael Dineen at the National Data Archive on Child Abuse and Neglect at Cornell University, has answered numerous questions for me about conducting child fatality-related research using the National Child Abuse and Neglect Data Set. He is patient, thoughtful, and always eager to help. The Center for the Advancement of Research and Scholarship at Bridgewater State University provided me with summer grants to further my research on fatal child maltreatment. This type of support for scholarship at a teaching-intensive university is unique and is just one example of the many ways that this university supports its faculty.

My husband has been a daily source of support for me: performing endless household tasks and listening to the vacillating stories of woe and excitement that come with being the partner of an academic in "book writing season." He is always patient and interested in helping me find a resolution to whatever problem I face. Finally, I must thank him for listening to some of the most heart-wrenching stories that exist: children dying from abuse or neglect at the hands of their caregivers. This goes beyond the "for better or for worse" contract, but he's handled it all with grace.

Contents

1 **Introduction to and Justification for the Book** 1
   References 7
2 **What Is Fatal Child Maltreatment?** 9
   2.1 What Constitutes Fatal Child Maltreatment? 10
   2.2 How Children Die 12
      2.2.1 Death by Physical Abuse 13
      2.2.2 Death by Neglect—Supervision 13
      2.2.3 Death by Neglect—Physical 15
      2.2.4 Death by Neglect—Medical 15
      2.2.5 Other and Multiple Forms of Maltreatment 16
   2.3 How Many Children Die? 16
   2.4 The Bottom Line 21
      2.4.1 What We Know 21
      2.4.2 What Remains Unknown 22
   References 22
3 **Risk Factors for Fatal Maltreatment Victimization and Perpetration** 27
   3.1 Commonly Accepted Risk Factors 28
      3.1.1 Child Age 28
      3.1.2 Child Gender 29
      3.1.3 Parent/Perpetrator Age 29
      3.1.4 Socioeconomic Status 29
      3.1.5 Household Risk Factors 30
   3.2 Areas of Controversy 31
      3.2.1 Perpetrator Characteristics 31
      3.2.2 Prior Involvement with Child Welfare/Social Services 32
      3.2.3 Race and Ethnicity of Victims and Perpetrators 33

		3.2.4	Child Behavior, Knowledge of Child Development, and the Parent-Child Relationship	35
	3.3	Unconfirmed Research		39
		3.3.1	Parent Mental Health	39
		3.3.2	Social Isolation	40
		3.3.3	Domestic Violence	40
		3.3.4	Child Disability Status	41
	3.4	The Bottom Line		41
		3.4.1	What We Know	41
		3.4.2	What Remains Unknown	42
	References			43
4	**The Intersection of the Child Welfare Profession and Maltreatment Fatalities**			47
	4.1	Child Maltreatment Fatalities: Perceptions and Experiences of Child Welfare Professionals Study		48
		4.1.1	CWWs' Knowledge, Practice Concerns, and Opinions About CMFs	48
		4.1.2	CWWs' Knowledge of Risk Factors for CMFs	50
		4.1.3	Training About CMFs	51
	4.2	Workers Who Experience the Death of a Child Client		53
		4.2.1	Handling of Case Prior to Fatality	55
		4.2.2	How Do Workers Miss Red Flags?	56
	4.3	The Aftermath of Child Maltreatment Fatalities		59
		4.3.1	Post-Traumatic Stress and Child Welfare	60
		4.3.2	Workers' Response to Experiencing a CMF	61
		4.3.3	Supporting Workers After a CMF	62
		4.3.4	Support Provided After Fatality	63
	4.4	The Bottom Line		64
		4.4.1	What We Know	64
		4.4.2	What Remains Unknown	65
	References			66
5	**Child Death Review Teams**			71
	5.1	Child Death Review Teams		71
	5.2	Purpose and Composition of CDRTs		72
	5.3	Selection Criteria and the Review Process		74
	5.4	Outputs of Child Death Review Teams		75
	5.5	Wide Acceptance and Use of Child Death Review Teams		77
	5.6	Outcomes of Child Death Review Teams: Controversy and Success		80
		5.6.1	Common Criticisms	80
		5.6.2	Lacking Evidence	81
		5.6.3	Bright Spots	83
	5.7	The Bottom Line		84
		5.7.1	What We Know	84

		5.7.2	What Remains Unknown	84
	References			87
6	**State Safe Haven Laws**		91
	6.1	The Problem of Abandoned and Discarded Infants	92
	6.2	History of Infant Abandonment and Safe Haven Laws	94
		6.2.1	The Specifics of Safe Haven Laws	95
	6.3	What if Safe Haven Laws Did Not Exist?	100
	6.4	Common Concerns About Safe Haven Laws	100
		6.4.1	Efficacy of Safe Haven Laws	100
		6.4.2	Too Little of the Wrong Thing, Too Late	101
		6.4.3	Marketing of Safe Haven Laws	103
		6.4.4	Rights of "Other" Parent	104
	6.5	The Bottom Line	104
		6.5.1	What We Know	104
		6.5.2	What Remains Unknown	105
	References			106
7	**Criminal Justice and Legal Reforms in Response to Fatal Child Maltreatment**		109
	7.1	The Scope of the Problem	110
		7.1.1	Problems with Investigations	110
		7.1.2	Limited Charges	111
		7.1.3	Problems Persist into the Courtroom	112
	7.2	Innovative Approaches at Multiple Levels	112
		7.2.1	Changes in Investigative Techniques	112
		7.2.2	Legal Responses to Increase Penalties for Child Abuse and Neglect Deaths	114
		7.2.3	Special Legal Reforms in Response to Religiously-Motivated Medical Child Maltreatment Fatalities	116
	7.3	Are Criminal Penalties Increasing?	118
	7.4	The Bottom Line	122
		7.4.1	What We Know	122
		7.4.2	What Remains Unknown	122
	References			123
8	**Prevention of Fatal Child Maltreatment: What Are We Doing That Is Working?**		127
	8.1	Levels of Prevention	127
	8.2	Previous Recommendations to Prevent Maltreatment Fatalities	128
	8.3	State and County Programs	128
	8.4	Prevention Programs That Are Specific to Fatal Child Maltreatment	129
		8.4.1	Shaken Baby Syndrome/Abusive Head Trauma	129
		8.4.2	Supervision of Children	132
		8.4.3	Safe Sleeping Environments for Children	135

	8.5	Prevention of Child Abuse and Neglect, in General	135
		8.5.1 Prevention Services	136
		8.5.2 Parenting Education	138
	8.6	The Bottom Line	140
		8.6.1 What We Know	140
		8.6.2 What Remains Unknown	141
		References	142

9 Conclusions and Recommendations Moving Forward in the Arena of Fatal Child Maltreatment 149

9.1	The Need for More and Better Research	149
	9.1.1 Incidence	150
	9.1.2 More Complete Data Sources	150
	9.1.3 Risk Factors	151
	9.1.4 CMFs and Helping Professions	152
9.2	What's Working?	153
9.3	Child Welfare Profession—Crisis or Crossroads?	155
9.4	What if We Focused on the *Fatal* Part of a Child Maltreatment Fatality?	157
9.5	Is There Any Good News?	158
9.6	What Are the Final Recommendations?	160
	References	161

Index 167

About the Author

Emily M. Douglas, Ph.D. is an associate professor of social work at Bridgewater State University in Bridgewater, Massachusetts. Her areas of expertise address child and family well being, and programs and policies that promote positive outcomes. Specifically, her areas of expertise include fatal child maltreatment, corporal punishment, partner violence, and divorced families. Dr. Douglas' interest in fatal child maltreatment began when she was in graduate school and worked for a child death review panel; it has remained a substantive research interest ever since. Her work in this area has focused on child death review teams, state policy, and the intersection of the child welfare profession and fatal maltreatment. Dr. Douglas has conducted the largest study on this issue, with over 425 child welfare professionals participating in a study about fatal maltreatment. She testified about this issue before the National Commission on the Elimination of Child Abuse and Neglect Fatalities in 2014. Dr. Douglas has also conducted research on male victims of female partner violence with her colleague, Dr. Denise Hines (Clark University); this research has been funded by the National Institutes of Health. Dr. Douglas has an undergraduate degree in psychology and graduate degrees in public policy; she also completed an NIMH-supported post-doctoral research fellowship under the mentorship of the late Dr. Murray Straus at the Family Research Laboratory at the University of New Hampshire. Dr. Douglas is the founder and director of the *National Research Conference on Child and Family Programs and Policy* which was held for five summers from 2008 to 2012. During the 2010–2011 academic year, Dr. Douglas was named the Presidential Fellow at Bridgewater State University, allowing her a full academic year to focus on her research on maltreatment fatalities and the child welfare system. Finally, Dr. Douglas is the author/co-author of three books on family policy issues and ~40 peer-reviewed publications; she also regularly presents at national and international conferences. At Bridgewater State University, she teaches courses in social policy, research methods, and directs the Graduate Writing Fellows program for the university campus. For the 2016–2017 academic year, Dr. Douglas will be a Congressional fellow in Washington, D.C. for the Society for Research on Child Development.

Chapter 1
Introduction to and Justification for the Book

As I sit down to write the introduction to this book, a mother from Blackstone, Massachusetts has been charged with the murder of two of three infants who were found deceased in a house that was filled with garbage, feces, rodents, and other vermin (see Text Box 1.1). A colleague just sent me a news story about a mother in Bastrop, Georgia, who left her two children, ages 3 and 4, unattended at home while she had her hair styled; a fire broke out and both children died (Text Box 1.2). A newspaper from upstate New York is reporting on the beating death of a toddler who was killed by his mother's boyfriend (Text Box 1.3). In 2014, a father in suburban Atlanta, Georgia area allegedly purposely killed his toddler by leaving him in a parked car while the father was at work; the boy died of heatstroke (Text Box 1.4). In Idaho, parents do not have to provide their children with healthcare if it is against their religious beliefs. There is an active faith-healing community in this state and children from that community are dying at a rate that is much higher than the rest of the population. In one religious community's cemetery, 25% of the graves are for children who have died—mostly from common, but untreated health conditions such as food poisoning, diabetes, infections, and the like (Text Box 1.5). This fall 2014, in Wisconsin, a father killed his 11-month old daughter by repeatedly throwing her to the ground and then tried to set his apartment on fire (Text Box 1.6).

Text Box 1.1
In Blackstone, Massachusetts, a 10-year-old boy was playing outside and asked a friend's mother how to get a baby to stop crying. That mother entered the boy's house to help out and found a 3-year-old in a crib with soiled diaper, covered with feces. In another room, she found an infant, also in a crib, crying and covered with feces. The house was knee-deep in trash, diapers, and human and animal feces. These three children and their 13-year-old sister were taken into the state's child protective agency. Upon examination, the 3-year-old was

(continued)

Text Box 1.1 (continued)
nutritionally deprived, had no muscle tone, and had maggots living in her ears. Law enforcement returned to the home the next day and found the skeletal remains of three infants and the carcasses of several animals. The mother and father both lived in the home. The father reported to have been banished to the basement and no knowledge of the four youngest children in the house or the deceased infants. The mother has been charged with two counts of murder (Moskowitz, 2014).

Text Box 1.2
A mother in Bastrop, Louisiana, left her two children ages 3 and 4, unattended while she had her hair styled. The children had no supervision and the house was being heated with space-heaters. A fire broke out in her absence and both of the children perished. The mother was charged with two counts of negligent homicide (Sommers, 2015).

Text Box 1.3
Shortly before a 2-year-old boy was beaten to death by his mother's male partner in upstate New York, the family had been reported to child protective services for suspected child maltreatment. The report was determined to be "unfounded" and the case was closed. Leading up to his death, the boy suffered several internal injuries and a head injury. His perpetrator has been indicted for second-degree murder (Pfeiffer, 2014).

Text Box 1.4
A father was pulled over on his way home from work, in suburban Atlanta, Georgia, wailing about his near 2-year-old son who he "found" in the backseat of his vehicle. The father told police that he accidentally left the child in the car when he was at work, but law enforcement found that the father had searched websites about living a "child free" life style and about animals dying in hot vehicles. The father has been charged with murder (Blinder, 2014; Fausset & Blinder, 2014).

Text Box 1.5
The Followers of Christ, who have an active faith community in Idaho, do not practice modern medicine. They believe that God's hand directs all human

(continued)

Text Box 1.5 (continued)
illness and that intervention is impure and is a sin. Like children in all communities, they are more vulnerable to illness than adults, and many of them have died from treatable conditions: food poisoning so severe that the child's esophagus ruptured; intestinal blockage; pneumonia; pre-mature delivery of an infant that had no pre-natal care; childhood diabetes; and a urinary tract infection. In one cemetery of the Followers of Christ, of the 553 marked graves, 144 are for minors; that's more than 25%. The laws in Idaho provide protection for parents who do not provide medical care because of their religious beliefs (Tilkin, 2013).

Text Box 1.6
An 11-month-old girl was killed by her father in Kenosha, Wisconsin. In what was reportedly a very violent attack, the father hit the mother, kicked her, and threw her down a set of stairs. The mother tried to escape with the infant, but the father caught up with them and grabbed the infant from her arms. He repeatedly threw the child on the ground, causing her death, just as a neighbor ran to intervene. The father ran back into their home and tried to set the apartment on fire. He told first responders that he wanted to kill his daughter to rid her of the evil inside of her, to destroy what he had created, and to save his daughter from the world (Luthern, 2014).

Children who die from abuse and neglect, or child maltreatment fatalities (CMFs) are the focus of this book. These victims are the subject of daily media reports and suffer the worst kind of outcome that results from abuse or neglect (Ayre, 2001; Cooper, 2005). The death of children is an upsetting topic; it's even more upsetting when children are killed; and, to be killed by the actions or inactions of one's parents moves into "the horrific." CMFs have increasingly received attention from scholars in the fields of child welfare, social work and human services, health, mental health, and law enforcement. Figure 1.1 shows the rapid increase in mentions of child deaths, in the context of abuse and neglect, in EBSCO databases (which is where scholarly, peer-reviewed publications are indexed) from 1970 to 2009.[1] I did not include years in the present decade in this quick search because we are only partially through this period of time, but from 2010 through the first month of 2015, there have already been 12,100 mentions of CMF-related content.

---

[1] I conducted a search for the terms "child death" AND "abuse OR neglect OR maltreatment." "Child death" had to be in the title; the other terms could appear anywhere in the search. It is my informal assessment that "child death" is used more frequently than "child fatality." Additionally, "child death" and "child fatality" are used interchangeably; thus, when I attempted to use both terms to conduct this search, many citations were double-counted.

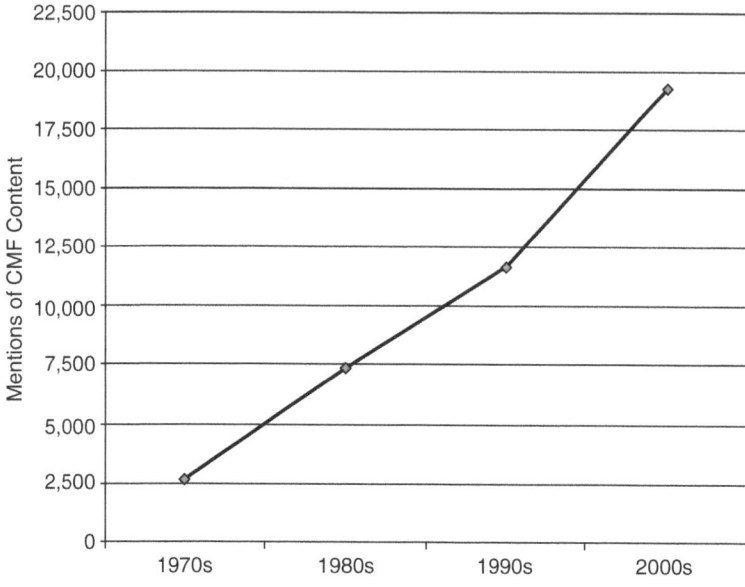

Figure 1.1 Mentions of Child Death with Child Abuse or Neglect in EBSCO Databases, 1970–2009

Over the past four-and-a-half decades, there have been many books dedicated to the topic of fatal child maltreatment, child homicide, infanticide, and the like. These books have primarily focused on describing the act of killing a child, the perpetrators and their relationships to the children, and the risk factors for perpetration and victimization. Some provide detailed information on the history of infanticide (Piers, 1978), including evolutionary rationales for the killing of infants (Hausfater & Hrdy, 1984). Other books have focused on all forms of child homicide, with each chapter outlining the perpetrators, motives, and culminating in the development of a theoretical understanding of child homicide (Adler & Polk, 2001; Alt & Wells, 2010; Schwartz & Isser, 2006) that is also accompanied by suggestions for prevention and intervention (Greenland, 1971). Still other books have focused exclusively on mothers and how maternal infanticide and child homicide are unique from all other forms of fatal maltreatment (McKee, 2006; Meyer, Oberman, & Rone, 2001; Oberman, 1996). These books primarily focus on the motivations for committing homicide and risk factors for identifying when a fatality might be imminent. All of these books have made important contributions to the professional literature and to the field's increased understanding about the circumstances under which children die and the potential reasons for why this happens.

The increase in attention from scholars has been paralleled, or surpassed by attention and activity on the ground by practitioners in these same fields: child welfare, social work, social services, health, mental health, and law enforcement. These actions, which have resulted in policies, programs, and other professional responses are part of larger policy responses that have aimed to protect children. The status of children as vulnerable, dependent on others, and whose development is influenced by their environments makes them prime candidates for special protections. (Garbarino, Hammond, Mercy, & Yung, 2004). For example, laws in the second half of the twentieth century have focused on providing children with appropriate non-family daycare (Butterfield, Rocha, & Butterfield, 2010; Zigler & Hall, 2000), protecting the best interests of the child in custody disputes (Goldstein, Freud, & Solnit, 1979; Goldstein, Freud, Solnit, & Burlingham, 1973; Goldstein, Freud, Solnit, & Goldstein, 1986; Skolnick, 2003), family-medical leave to support new and sick children (Brown, 2009), and have established our modern-day child welfare system (Gelles, 1996).

Those policies and programs that are focused on reducing or eliminating CMFs are the focus of this book. Only one other set of books has focused on the larger systemic responses to fatal child maltreatment, and that was a two-part series that examined multidisciplinary workgroups that reviewed the deaths of children in several Western nations (Vincent, 2010a, 2010b). In the following pages, I outline the history, and the varied responses from different professional groups, along with the outcomes of those responses. My focus is on whether these responses are successful which is measured by whether fewer children die as a result of these efforts. This particular angle is what distinguishes this book from other approaches and publications that already exist. Thus, each chapter will conclude with what I call "the bottom line" regarding our knowledge of each response to fatal child abuse and neglect, where I highlight what we *know* and what we *do not know* about CMFs. Summaries and conclusions of each chapter are reserved for the final chapter of the book. Additionally, it is also my attempt to make CMFs and the complexities of their cases real to the reader, thus I have provided examples of CMFs and our responses to this problem throughout the book.

Not surprisingly, there are different camps of thought regarding the effectiveness of most of the approaches that I review in this book. Therefore, I address each approach by noting the areas of controversy within. In fact, I begin each chapter with an overview of the controversy concerning the selected policy, program, or other professional response, so that readers can orient themselves to the different ideological or theoretical approaches. Compared with other research I have conducted, such as on male victims of partner violence, parental use of corporal punishment, and the role of fathers in parenting post-divorce, the controversies that I highlight may not seem especially contentious. Colleagues who read and provided feedback on chapters in this book mentioned in passing, "This doesn't seem very heated as some other topics in the social sciences!" Indeed, that may be the case. But, the arguments that are presented here—such as whether an intoxicated parent who co-sleeps with an infant and then accidentally smothers the child could be substantiated for neglect, or whether laws that allow desperate parents to legally relinquish a newborn take our attention away from universal contraception or promoting relinquishment through traditional adoption—are at the heart of what we consider to be fatal child maltreatment and how we try to prevent it. They are not highly politicized arguments that are played out in the media, but for those in the field, these controversies are the points of contention that are debated and have important implications for how we categorize, count, understanding and thus, try to prevent instances of children's deaths.

Throughout this book, I will introduce a number of different terms and approaches; I will define those as I go through each policy, program, or professional response. But, allow me to introduce two of the more routinely used concepts here, as they appear throughout the book.

- Child maltreatment fatality—"an injury resulting from the abuse and neglect was the cause of death; or abuse and neglect were contributing factors to the cause of death" (U.S. Department of Health & Human Services, 2012, p. 118)
- Levels of prevention—Throughout this book I also discuss levels of prevention, as the field of public health defines them (Centers for Disease Control and Prevention, 2007):
  - Primary prevention is preventing a problem because it occurs, such as among the general population;
  - Secondary prevention is preventing a problem among those who are at risk for that problem; and,
  - Tertiary prevention is preventing the re-occurrence of a problem once it has surfaced and been treated.

This book has two primary areas: (1) defining and understanding risk factors for fatal child maltreatment to set the stage for thinking about prevention; and (2) reviewing and exploring the efficacy of multiple responses to CMFs. They are briefly explained here.

Chapter 2 provides definitions of fatal child maltreatment and explains why it is so difficult to provide accurate prevalence rates of CMFs. Chapter 3 focuses on risk factors for CMFs, which include child, parent, and household risk factors, as well as the parent-child relationship. In this chapter, I also outline the dearth of information concerning the distinction between fatal and non-fatal maltreatment.

Chapters 4, 5, 6, 7, and 8 turn to the heart of this book, which is to examine the policy, program, and other professional responses to fatal child maltreatment. I begin this section with the most and least obvious response: Chapter 4 focuses on the child welfare profession, their preparation for preventing CMFs, how they survive the aftermath of a child dying on caseload, and I speculate as to why workers miss red flags. Child welfare workers are in the business of preventing fatalities and this chapter addresses what might keep workers from being able to do this part of their job. Chapter 5 addresses one of the most popular responses to instances of fatal child maltreatment. Child death review teams (CDRTs) are multidisciplinary workgroups that examine the characteristics of children who die and seek to identify gaps in the system that may have failed to provide an adequate safety net for children. CDRTs exist in every state in the nation and are the only approach to CMFs that bring together different professional groups to sit at the same table to talk about their approaches to working with children and their families. Chapter 6 focuses on safe haven laws, which allow parents to legally relinquish new infants at designated locations without fear of criminal prosecution. Safe haven laws also exist in every state in the nation; they offer a last minute solution to parents who are feeling desperate about parenting a new child. Chapter 7 is dedicated to addressing the criminal justice responses to CMFs, such as changing the laws so that perpetrators can be more harshly punished for taking the life of a child than previously standing laws permitted. This chapter also addresses changes that have been made in state statute concerning the ability to criminally prosecute parents who have not provided medical treatment for their children due to their own religious beliefs. In the final response to CMFs, Chapter 8 focuses on programs that might prevent CMFs. There are no programs that specifically focus on CMFs, but many focus on targeted types of maltreatment, such as shaken baby syndrome, or abuse and neglect in general. The final part of this book is Chapter 9, which brings together themes that emerged across the chapters; I present the strongest conclusions about what works, what does not work, what additional information we need, and I make recommendations for moving forward.

References

Adler, C., & Polk, K. (2001). *Child victims of homicide*. Cambridge, UK: Cambridge University Press.

Alt, B. L., & Wells, S. K. (2010). *When caregivers kill: Understanding child murder by parents and other guardians*. Lanham, MD: Rowman & Littlefield.

Ayre, P. (2001). Child protection and the media: Lessons from the last three decades. *British Journal of Social Work, 31*(6), 887–901.

Blinder, A. (2014, September 4). Father charged with murder in hot-car death, and death penalty is weighed. *The New York Times*. Retrieved from http://www.nytimes.com/2014/09/05/us/father-charged-with-murder-in-death-of-boy-in-hot-car.html?_r=0

Brown, M. (2009). The 'state' of paid family leave: Insights from the 2006 & 2007 legislative sessions. In E. M. Douglas (Ed.), *Innovations in child and family policy: Multidisciplinary research and perspectives on strengthening children and their families*. Lanham, MD: Lexington Books.

Butterfield, A. K., Rocha, C. J., & Butterfield, W. H. (2010). *The dynamics of family policy: Analysis and advocacy*. Chicago, IL: Lyceum.

Centers for Disease Control and Prevention. (2007). Module 13: Levels of disease prevention. *EXCITE – Skin cancer module: Practice exercises*. Retrieved March 27, 2013, from http://www.cdc.gov/excite/skincancer/mod13.htm#levels

Cooper, L. (2005). Implications of media scrutiny for a child protection agency. *Journal of Sociology and Social Welfare, 32*(3), 107–121.

Fausset, R., & Blinder, A. (2014, July 11). Examining a father's role in a toddler's death. *The New York Times*. Retrieved from http://www.nytimes.com/2014/07/12/us/friends-and-prosecutors-deconstruct-fathers-role-in-toddlers-death.html

Garbarino, J., Hammond, W. R., Mercy, J., & Yung, B. R. (2004). Community violence and children: Preventing exposure and reducing harm. In K. I. Maton, C. J. Schellenbach, S. Leadbetter, & A. L. Solarz (Eds.), *Investing in children, youth, families, and communities*. Washington, DC: American Psychological Association.

Gelles, R. J. (1996). *The book of David: How preserving families can cost children's lives*. New York, NY: Basic Books.

Goldstein, J., Freud, A., & Solnit, A. J. (1979). *Before the best interests of the child*. New York, NY: Free Press.

Goldstein, J., Freud, A., Solnit, A. J., & Burlingham, D. (1973). *Beyond the best interests of the child*. New York, NY: Free Press.

Goldstein, J., Freud, A., Solnit, A. J., & Goldstein, S. (1986). *In the best interests of the child.* New York, NY: Free Press.

Greenland, C. (1971). Violence and dangerous behaviour associated with mental illness: Prospects for prevention. *Canadian Journal of Criminology and Corrections, 13*(4), 331–339.

Hausfater, G., & Hrdy, S. B. (Eds.). (1984). *Infanticide: Comparative and evolutionary perspectives.* New York, NY: Aldine Publishing Company.

Luthern, A. (2014, November 20). Kenosha dad charged with homicide in beating death of baby girl. *Journal Sentinel.* Retrieved from http://www.jsonline.com/news/babyhomi21-b99394707z1-283387941.html

McKee, G. R. (2006). *Why mothers kill: A forensic psychologist's casebook.* New York, NY: Oxford University Press.

Meyer, C., Oberman, M., & Rone, M. (2001). *Mothers who kill their children: Understanding the acts of moms from Susan Smith to the "prom mom".* New York, NY: New York University Press.

Moskowitz, E. (2014, December 29). Horrors Blackstone police allegedly found detailed in court. *The Boston Globe.* Retrieved from http://www.bostonglobe.com/metro/2014/12/29/blackstone-woman-due-worcester-courtroom-murder-children/2uVxaviOF6ANPDmNPjDmtN/story.html

Oberman, M. (1996). Mothers who kill: Coming to terms with modern American infanticide. *American Criminal Law Review, 34*, 1.

Pfeiffer, M. B. (2014, December 20). Care of Mason DeCosmo, 2, probed before abuse death. *Poughkeepsie Journal.* Retrieved from http://www.poughkeepsiejournal.com/story/news/local/2014/12/20/mason-decosmo-child-abuse-kenneth-stahli-katlin-wolfert/20704183/

Piers, M. W. (1978). *Infanticide: Past and present.* New York, NY: W.W. Norton & Company Inc.

Schwartz, L. L., & Isser, K. K. (2006). *Child homicide: Parents who kill.* New York, NY: CRC Press.

Skolnick, A. (2003). Soloman's children: The new biologism, psychological parenthood, attachment theory, and the best interests standard. In M. A. Mason, A. Skolnick, & S. D. Sugarman (Eds.), *All our families: New policies for a new century* (2nd ed., pp. 285–305). Oxford, NY: Oxford University Press.

Sommers, C. (2015, January 14). Police: Kids, left alone die in house fire while mother is out getting hair done. *CNN.* Retrieved from http://www.cnn.com/2015/01/14/us/louisiana-children-house-fire/index.html

Tilkin, D. (2013, November 7). Fallen followers: Investigation finds 10 mire dead children of faith healers. *KATU-TV.* Retrieved from http://www.katu.com/news/investigators/Fallen-followers-Investigation-finds-10-more-dead-children-of-faith-healers-231050911.html

U.S. Department of Health & Human Services. (2012). *Child maltreatment 2011: Reports from the States to the National Child Abuse and Neglect Data Systems – National statistics on child abuse and neglect.* Washington, DC: Administration for Children & Families, U.S. Department of Health & Human Services.

Vincent, S. (2010a). *Learning from child deaths and serious abuse.* Edinburgh, UK: Dunedin Academic Press Ltd.

Vincent, S. (2010b). *Preventing child deaths: Learning from review.* Edinburgh, UK: Dunedin Academic Press Ltd.

Zigler, E. F., & Hall, N. W. (2000). *Child development and social policy.* New York, NY: McGraw Hill.

Chapter 2
What Is Fatal Child Maltreatment?

What is fatal maltreatment? At first it seems like a simple question—instances of abuse or neglect where children die. At the broadest level, it is simple, but in the particular, it is complex: a 3-year old who is left alone by his mother wanders into traffic and is hit by a car and killed; a 5-year old is kicked in the stomach by her mother's boyfriend—her intestines rupture and she dies; an infant's head is smashed into a wall by a father; an 18-month old falls into a bucket of toxic liquid and drowns while a caregiver is on the phone; an infant is found dead in her intoxicated parents' bed; a mother forgets her sleeping infant is in the car with her on a warm, sunny day and leaves him unattended for 5 hours—he is deceased when he is discovered by a neighbor; a 2-year old child finds a bottle of Benadryl pills and, thinking that it is candy, eats the whole bottle; or a 2-year old falls from an unsecured window while a parent sleeps in the neighboring room.

In the introductory chapter, I explained that the controversies in the professional fields that deal with fatal child abuse neglect will be highlighted throughout the book. The present chapter, which explores definitions of fatal maltreatment and prevalence rates, is nothing but controversy; the issues addressed in this chapter primarily focus on two overarching issues:

- How we define fatal maltreatment varies not only by state, but by county and sometimes by medical examiner.
- When our definitions vary by locality, it can be difficult to count how often something happens. Further, when we change how we define something, it can have an immediate effect on how it is counted.

The primary purpose of this chapter is to provide an introduction to the topic of fatal maltreatment and to set the stage for getting into the meat of this book, which is the examination of policies, programs, and professional responses to deaths resulting from child abuse or neglect.

Text Box 2.1

Quoted from the *Miami Herald*, August 2013: "One by one, Florida Sen. Eleanor Sobel read the names or initials of 20 children — children who died this summer while on the radar of the state's embattled child welfare agency. Some were beaten savagely. Others suffocated or drowned. One was strangled, and another run over by a car. The listing of the dead was a dramatic way to launch a town hall meeting designed to bring reforms and save lives" (Miller & Burch, 2013).

2.1 What Constitutes Fatal Child Maltreatment?

The controversies around fatal child maltreatment begin with what we call it. The professional literature on death by child abuse and neglect encompasses many different terms: child maltreatment fatality (CMF), child abuse death, neonaticide, infanticide, filicide, child homicide, parental homicide, and child murder encompass most of the terms that are used. To the public at large, the differences between these terms is likely not important; the public is generally most concerned that a child has died at the hands of a caregiver, as opposed to the classification of death (see Text Boxes 2.1 and 2.2). But, these different terms have salience within the professional literature, largely due to the measurement or tracking of the problem or because of criminal justice responses. Some definitions of these terms follow:

- The Bureau of Justice Statistics defines *homicide* as: "…murder and non-negligent manslaughter, which is the willful killing of one human being by another" (U.S. Bureau of Justice Statistics, n.d.). Statistics often reference *child homicide* or *homicide against children*. The categories of age vary considerably, but where abuse and neglect are concerned, victims are likely to be very young, generally under the age of 5 (U.S. Department of Health & Human Services, 2012) (see Chapter 3 for more information on age).
- The terms *neonaticide*, *infanticide*, and *filicide* refer to killing children of differing ages and the killing of children by family members. There is little disagreement that *neonaticide* refers to killing a child within the first few days of life (McKee, 2006). *Infanticide* has been referred to as the killing of a child under the age of 1 year (McKee, 2006); the organization Child Trends, however, calls this *infant homicide* (Child Trends, 2012). To further complicate matters, the U.S. Bureau of Justice Statistics defines infanticide as the killing of a child under the age of 5 (Fox & Zawitz, 2004). *Filicide* is not a term that is used in official crime statistics, but scholars have referred to this as the killing of children older than 1 year of age (McKee, 2006) or more broadly, the killing of a child by his or her parent or parents (Adler & Polk, 2001).

2.1 What Constitutes Fatal Child Maltreatment?

Most of these terms apply specifically to children who died from abuse, as opposed to neglect. Instances of neglect do not always meet the legal standard for homicide. For example, when a parent leaves his child in a vehicle for hours instead of providing supervision and the child dies, or a child falls from an unsecure location, or a parent does not seek medical care for a child because of the family's religious beliefs, it is difficult to prove that these are instances that meet the definition of homicide, "willful killing of one human being by another" (Bureau of Justice Statistics, 2014). I spend more time on legal definitions and responses to fatal maltreatment in Chapter 7. In this book, I cast a wide net and focus on children's deaths that result from both abuse and neglect. I will primarily use the term child maltreatment fatality or CMF.

- The U.S. Child Abuse and Prevention Act, first enacted in 1974, includes death in its definition of child abuse and neglect: "Any recent act or failure to act on the part of a parent or caretaker, which results in death, serious physical or emotional harm, sexual abuse, or exploitation, or an act or failure to act which presents an imminent risk of serious harm" (U.S. Children's Bureau, 2011).
- The National Child Abuse and Neglect Data System (NCANDS), on which annual U.S. rates of maltreatment are based, states that a death is classified as a child maltreatment fatality or a child abuse and neglect death "because either an injury resulting from the abuse and neglect was the cause of death; or abuse and neglect were contributing factors to the cause of death" (U.S. Department of Health & Human Services, 2012).

Not surprisingly, there is considerable overlap in the professional literature and in prevention efforts that focus on CMFs and homicide by parents. Thus, I draw from all of the literature on abuse and neglect-related deaths, regardless of legal definitions.

Text Box 2.2

- In 2011: A nearly 2-year-old boy died in Massachusetts after falling from his open bedroom window while his mother slept; the home was described as trash-ridden and almost uninhabitable (Murray, 2011).
- In 2011: A 5-month-old infant girl died in Massachusetts after taking a bottle of formula laced with heroin (Ellement, 2013).
- In 2012: A 22-month-old child who was locked in her bedroom by her mother for days at a time with her siblings died from malnutrition and dehydration in Texas (Davis, 2013).
- In 2013: A 12-year-old boy died in Georgia from an apparent beating. He had multiple bruises, human bite marks, lacerations, and other marks consistent with physical abuse (Stevens, 2013).

2.2 How Children Die

The United States Administration for Children and Families, of the Department of Health and Human Services, publishes an annual report concerning the abuse and neglect of children and the services that they receive. The information contained in this report, simply titled *Child Maltreatment,* comes from information that is gathered by each state's child welfare information system and is reported to the federal government. That data is the basis for NCANDS, which is released annually and is housed at the National Data Archive for Child Abuse & Neglect at Cornell University, and is available to the public. The federal government also uses this data, which is aggregated, analyzed, and published in an annual report: *Child Maltreatment.*[1] The first *Child Maltreatment* report that contained information about children dying from maltreatment was in 1996. For over the past decade, Chapter 4 of this annual report has been dedicated to fatalities. The most recently available report at the time of writing this chapter is information from 2014. These reports always show that children are more likely to die from neglect than physical abuse. When averaged together, information from 2010 to 2014 shows that of CMF victims, 79 % died of neglect and 45 % died of physical abuse (U.S. Department of Health & Human Services, 2011–2015). The percentage of deaths sums to more than 100 % because as many as one-third of CMF victims die of multiple forms of maltreatment (U.S. Department of Health & Human Services, 2010). The media tends to focus on deaths from abuse much more than deaths from neglect, in large measure because they are more dramatic stories (i.e., shaking a baby versus a baby suffocating while co-sleeping with an intoxicated parent) and because abuse cases are more likely to be criminally prosecuted (Liang & Macfarlane, 1999). This is probably why child welfare workers are more likely to think that more children die from abuse than neglect (Douglas, 2012).

Even though more children die from neglect, the rates at which victims of abuse or neglect die differs. I used information from the *Child Maltreatment* reports containing data from 2009 to 2013 and found that for every 1,000 children suffering from medical neglect, 6.93 die; for every 1,000 children suffering from physical neglect, 1.65 children die; and, for every 1,000 children suffering from physical abuse, 4.79 die. When the medical neglect and physical neglect are combined into one category, the rate is 1.81 per 1,000 children already suffering from neglect. In order to calculate this, I used the sources of information that permitted multiple count of different types of maltreatment per victim. Thus, even though more children die from neglect, this is directly related to the fact that neglect is more prevalent than abuse. The relative risk for each type of maltreatment differs substantially, with medical neglect being the most risky for children.

What's most important to remember about causes of children's deaths by maltreatment is that the causes do not differ from non-fatal maltreatment. When a death

---

[1] Individuals can gain access to the annual reports by visiting the U.S. Children's Bureau website of the U.S. Administration for Children & Families; they have a page that is dedicated to the *Child Maltreatment* reports, http://www.acf.hhs.gov/programs/cb/research-data-technology/statistics-research/child-maltreatment.

2.2 How Children Die

is involved, it means that the abuse or neglect was more extreme than what generally occurs in instances of non-fatal maltreatment. With some exception (see Chapter 7), state statutes do not have definitions of fatal child maltreatment that differ from definitions of non-fatal child maltreatment. Physical abuse is the same whether a child lives or dies and the same is true for all other forms of maltreatment. When a child dies, the same standards are applied to determine if maltreatment was involved as if the child had survived. Text Box 2.2 provides some examples of actual cases where children have died from abuse and/or neglect. Readers will note that the conditions under which children die from maltreatment are extremely varied. Table 2.1 provides detailed causes of deaths that a child might experience; the causes of death are listed in alphabetical order.

2.2.1 Death by Physical Abuse

Children's deaths by means of physical abuse primarily take the form of beatings, blunt-force trauma, and abusive head trauma—which is a broader category of what the public generally calls "shaken baby syndrome." Abusive head trauma is one of the primary ways that very young children die from physical abuse (Klevens & Leeb, 2010; Palusci & Covington, 2014). Some of the causes of death that are less well known and warrant explanation include immersion burns and medical child abuse. In these instances, the perpetrator "dips" a child in boiling or scalding-hot water, such as in a bathtub—usually as a form of discipline. Children do not usually immediately die as a result of immersion burns, but can later die as a result of dehydration or infection resulting from the burns (Young & Hyden, 2003). Deaths that result from medical child abuse or factitious disorder by proxy (formerly called Munchausen syndrome by proxy) occur when a caregiver creates medical conditions or medical crises for his or her child by making the child sick or stopping the child's breathing, in an attempt to gain attention for him or herself (Flaherty, 2013; Mash, Frazier, Nowacki, Worley, & Goldfarb, 2011; Stirling, Abuse, & Neglect, 2007; Tsai et al., 2012). This form of child abuse has been featured in the media and has been the subject of a made-for-TV movie, *A Child's Cry for Help*, but is not a common form of child maltreatment (Schreier & Libow, 1993). The other causes of death that are listed as a form of physical abuse in Table 2.1 are primarily self-explanatory.

2.2.2 Death by Neglect—Supervision

Most of the children who die from neglect die from a lack of supervision or when a parent has failed to protect his or her child from harm (Palusci & Covington, 2014). When children die from neglect, they are most likely to die around sources of water,

Table 2.1 Potential Causes of Death Due to Child Maltreatment

Examples of Physical Abuse

- Abusive head trauma—*shaking an infant, hitting infant's head on hard surface*
- Blunt force trauma—*beating, kicking, punching, throwing against floor, wall, ceiling*
- Medical child abuse/Factitious disorder by proxy (formerly called Munchausen syndrome by proxy)—*deliberately causing illness/injury in an effort to gain personal attention/sympathy*
- Immersion burns—*submerging child (or portion of body) into hot water (or other liquid)*
- Immersive drowning—*purposely drowning child*
- Poisoning—*purposely poisoning child or giving too much medication*
- Stabbing/shooting—*purposely stabbing or shooting a child*
- Suffocation/strangulation—*purposely suffocating or strangling a child*

Examples of Neglect

Supervisory	Physical	Medical
• Animal bites—*inadequate supervisory around dangerous animals* • Driving under the influence—*while children are in vehicle* • Drowning—*inadequate supervisory around sources of water/liquid* • Falls—*inadequate supervisory around heights (i.e., windows)* • Firearm discharge—*inadequate supervisory around firearm* • Hit by car—*inadequate supervisory around roadways* • House fire—*inadequate supervisory around fire materials, or leaving children alone where fire starts* • Left in car—*purposely leaving child in car unsupervised* • Ingestion/poisoning—*inadequate supervisory around poisonous substances* • Suffocation—*unsafe sleeping environments*	• Exposure to elements—*abandoning an infant or young child (e.g., newborn in toilet), leaving child outside in cold or heat without adequate protection* • Malnutrition, starvation, failure-to-thrive—*providing inadequate nutrition for child* • Unsafe housing conditions—*living in a home which is not up-to-code* • Unsanitary conditions—*living conditions that are unsanitary and unhealthy*	• Failure to seek treatment—*failure to seek medical treatment for a sick or injured child* • Failure to comply with treatment—*failure to comply with medical treatment which has been recommended or ordered* • Refusal of treatment—*refusing to comply with medical treatment which has been recommended or ordered*

specifically in the bathroom of their home. In such instances, very young children are left alone in bathtubs or under the "supervision" of other young siblings (Margolin, 1990). Small children can also fall into pools or into buckets with fluid in them. Over the past decade there has been increased attention from the media, child welfare, and legal professionals about leaving young children unsupervised in automobiles; these cases often involve warm temperatures so that children are at an increased risk of overheating while trapped inside (McLaren, Null, & Quinn, 2005). Another area concerning child death, which has received increased attention, is safe sleeping environments for children. Suffocation and strangulation due to unsafe sleeping environments has been on the increase over the past several decades (Shapiro-Mendoza, Kimball, Tomashek, Anderson, & Blanding, 2009); see Chapter 8 for more information on these topics. Children can also fall to their death—out of windows without screens or balconies lacking adequate safeguards (Harris, Rochette, & Smith, 2011). Textbox 2.2 describes a child who fell from a third-floor window while his mother slept; he died several days later. The home did not have screens in the windows and there was furniture stacked by the window, which made it possible for the toddler to climb and reach the window. The home was also filled with trash and debris so that it was nearly impossible for an adult to walk through the apartment (Murray, 2011). Table 2.1 lists additional ways that children can die from a lack of supervision.

2.2.3 *Death by Neglect—Physical*

The most prominent cases of physical neglect have involved women who abandon newborns in public places (Meyer, Oberman, & Rone, 2001). These stories have involved women who did not know that they were pregnant or did not share their pregnancy with anyone else. Many of the stories have involved abandoning infants in toilets, on bathroom floors, in dumpsters, and the like; see Chapter 6 for more information on this topic. In other circumstances of physical neglect, children can be purposely starved to death. Textbox 2.2 depicts a case where a child was routinely locked in a bedroom for days at a time without adequate nutrition; she died from malnutrition and dehydration. Children's physical environments can result in fatal outcomes, such as a child living in a home with piles of trash because of hoarding, animal or human feces on the floors, or when a home is not up-to-code, thus leaving a child vulnerable to exposed wires, unsafe floorboards, and the like.

2.2.4 *Death by Neglect—Medical*

Children die as a result of medical neglect, which can take several different forms. One, parents may fail to seek medical treatment because they have caused an injury to their child and they fear losing their child to child protective services or potential criminal prosecution. Two, parents may seek medical attention, but fail or refuse to comply with the recommendations/orders of health professionals. This may be related to philosophical or religious beliefs, a fear of treatment (i.e., parents do not want their children taking medicine), or because the parent's capacity to parent is limited due to circumstances in their own lives, such as struggling with addiction, cognitive limitations, mental health concerns, or lack of knowledge of child development (Berkowitz, 2003). Third, many parents who fail to seek medical treatment or comply with health orders do so for religious reasons. Some religions do not endorse or support the use of modern medicine. In such instances, the few parents who seek medical attention for their children are shamed for failing to be "holy enough" to save their children through prayer and can be banned from the church upon a child's death. The most mainstream religion with these views is Christian Science (Asser & Swan, 1998; Swan, 1997); see Chapters 3 and 7 for more information on this topic.

2.2.5 Other and Multiple Forms of Maltreatment

A very small percentage of children also die from sexual abuse. In 2014, 1.1% of CMF victims died as a result of this form of abuse (U.S. Department of Health & Human Services, 2015). In such instances children sustain life-threatening injuries as a result of the sexual abuse; this is especially true for very young children, such as infants, who may be the victim of a rape, which can cause significant injuries (Pitcher & Bowley, 2002).

As noted already, children can die from multiple forms of maltreatment. A child could suffer a blunt force trauma to the body and then be medically neglected so that she dies as a result of both forms of maltreatment: physical abuse and failure to seek medical treatment. Further, children who die from maltreatment are often subjected to multiple forms of maltreatment even if only one type is the cause of death. For example, children who are physically assaulted are likely to suffer emotional or psychological abuse at the same time. Even though the issue of dying from multiple forms of maltreatment is known and is recognized annually in federal reports (U.S. Department of Health & Human Services, 2015), there has been virtually no research which has examined or compared children who have died solely from a single form of abuse or neglect with children who have died from multiple forms of maltreatment. This is just one of the areas where there is a tremendous need for additional research.

2.3 How Many Children Die?

The rate at which children die, from all causes, has drastically dropped over the last century, in the United States and across the globe. For example, between 1915 and 1997, the infant mortality rate dropped from 100 per 100 live births to 7 (Centers

2.3 How Many Children Die?

for Disease Control, 1999). A similar decline, among children under the age of 5, was noted in western European nations during this timeframe (Corsini & Viazzo, 1993). According to the World Health Organization, from 1955 through the 1990s, there was a 17.5% decline in child mortality rates throughout the world (Ahmad, Lopez, & Inoue, 2000). Despite many regional differences, between 1990 and 2015 alone, the child mortality rate for children under the age of 5 has dropped 53% worldwide (United Nations Children's Fund, 2015). These changes are the result of wide-scale improvements in many areas: environmental regulation, nutrition, medicine, access to healthcare, monitoring of diseases, consumer product safety, education, and overall standard of living (Centers for Disease Control, 1999).

The number of children who die from abuse or neglect each year, however, is a source of significant controversy (Finkelhor & Jones, 2012). The 2014 *Child Maltreatment* report shows that in that year, 1,580 children died from maltreatment and that between 2010 and 2014, an average of 1,574 children died each year (U.S. Department of Health & Human Services, 2015). Figure 2.1 plots the number of children who died from maltreatment in the U.S., as well as the rate of CMFs from 1996 to 2012. Specifically, on the right vertical axis is the total number of children who died from maltreatment each year. On the left vertical axis is the rate of children who died from maltreatment. Tragic as they are, CMFs happen so infrequently that they have to be calculated as the number of children who die per 100,000 living children in the U.S. The figure easily displays a rapid increase in the number and rate of CMFs over the last near-two decades: starting at 1.68 CMFs per 100,000

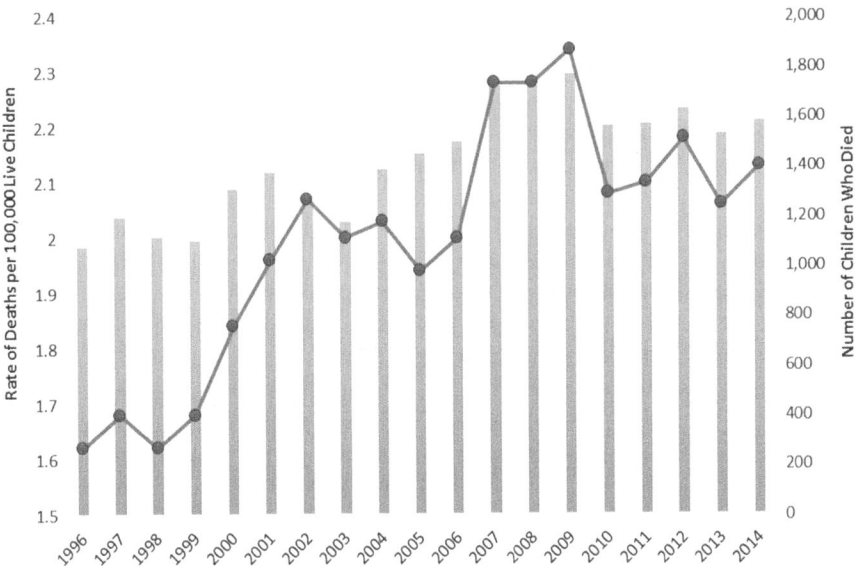

Figure 2.1 Number and Rate of Fatal Child Maltreatment in the United States 1996–2011 (*Source: U.S. Department of Health & Human Services*)

children in 1996 and peaking at 2.34 in 2009, despite the fact that this was during a time when child fatalities was on the decline, overall (Murphy, Xu, & Kochanek, 2013). In 2014, the rate was 2.13 per 100,000 live children (U.S. Department of Health & Human Services, 2015).

These rates are high compared to other European and western nations. The World Health Organization reported the annual child homicide rates among children under 15 years of age, for 40 different countries for the period of 2006–2010 (Sethi et al., 2013). The statistics are not directly comparable to U.S. numbers because the age range only goes up to 15, as opposed to 18 in the U.S. and even though the report indicates that all of the perpetrators were parents or caregivers, it is not clear how many deaths attributed to neglect are included. Using the information in the report, I calculated the average homicide rate among children up to age 15, with parent/caregiver perpetrators, for these 40 nations to be 0.45 per 100,000 live children. The report also contains deaths due to undetermined intent, which is a common reporting technique when handling international CMF rates (UNICEF, 2003). When child maltreatment deaths due to known homicides are combined with child deaths due to undetermined intent, the rate is 0.77 per 100,000 live children (Sethi et al., 2013), which is still only one-third of the rate in the United States.

This apparent increase in CMFs has been the subject of significant scrutiny. Many have questioned whether CMFs could actually increase during a time when other forms of maltreatment, namely, physical and sexual abuse declined in the U.S. (Child Maltreatment Research Listserv, 2009; Finkelhor, Jones, & Shattuck, 2010; Jones & Finkelhor, 2003; Jones, Finkelhor, & Halter, 2006). At the same time, the field has openly acknowledged that children's deaths due to maltreatment have been under-recognized and thus, undercounted for years both in the U.S. and other rich nations (UNICEF, 2003). CMFs have often erroneously been identified as cases of accidental suffocation/injury, sudden infant/unexpected death syndrome (SIDS/SUDS), or deaths due to undetermined/unknown causes (Ewigman, Kivlahan, & Land, 1993; Herman-Giddens et al., 1999; Soerdjbalie-Maikoe, Bilo, van den Akker, & Maes, 2010; Tursz, Crost, Gerbouin-Rerolle, & Cook, 2010). Even today, in the U.S. and throughout Europe, medical examiners struggle to give accurate determinations regarding causes of death, especially among infants (Kim, Shapiro-Mendoza, Chu, Camperlengo, & Anderson, 2012; Sethi et al., 2013), who are most likely to be victims of CMFs (U.S. Department of Health & Human Services, 2015). In Missouri fewer than half of children who died from maltreatment in the mid-1980s had deaths that were accurately classified as related to abuse or neglect (Ewigman et al., 1993). Similar results were found in North Carolina with a retrospective analysis of deaths between 1985 and 1994—61% of maltreatment deaths were incorrectly classified (Herman-Giddens et al., 1999). Some estimate that the actual number of CMFs in the U.S. could be as high as 5,000 each year (United States Advisory Board on Child Abuse and Neglect, 1995), but official statistics have usually come in around 1,500–1,700 each year.

Even in the face of poor classification regarding the causes of death, there have been important changes in how child deaths are investigated, primarily in the legal and medical fields, in an effort to more accurately identify CMF cases (see Chapter

7) (Dallas Police Department, 1994; Garstang & Sidebotham, 2008; Herman-Giddens et al., 1999; Lanning & Walsh, 1996; Levene & Bacon, 2004). For example, the American Academy of Pediatrics has issued and re-issued guidelines regarding how to determine if a child's death is attributable to intentional suffocation versus SIDS/SUDS and how to handle grieving caregivers, whether they are "guilty" or not (Committee on Child Abuse and Neglect-American Academy of Pediatrics, 1994; Hymel & Committee on Child Abuse and Neglect-American Academy of Pediatrics, 2006; Pediatrics, 2001). Further, as causes of death from SID/SUDS have fallen, recent attention has turned to deaths due to accidental suffocation and strangulation in bed (ASSB) (Gilchrist, Ballesteros, & Parker, 2012; Shapiro-Mendoza et al., 2009). Between 1984 and 2004, deaths due to ASSB increased by more than a factor of 4, from 2.8 to 12.5 per 100,000 live births (Shapiro-Mendoza et al., 2009). The professional literature (Kim et al., 2012) and practitioners in the field have offered anecdotal evidence which suggests that the line between ruling a child's death SIDS/SUDS, ASSB, suffocation (intentional or not), or unknown, is fluid and that there is significant disagreement between practitioners, sometimes even within the same region. Given these circumstances, it is very difficult to capture an accurate statistic concerning the rate of CMFs in the U.S., especially among infants.

As a way to try to get a handle on these changes, new federal legislation in the United States mandates that states provide information on the sources of data that states use and do *not use* to count and report cases of fatal child maltreatment ("Child and Family Services Improvement and Innovation Act," 2011; National Conference of State Legislatures, 2011). States also have to submit a proposal for how they plan to gather data from additional sources in the future. For example, states are encouraged to gather information from their child welfare information systems, child death review teams (CDRTs) (See Chapter 5 for more information), medical examiner/coroner's office, and the like. The thinking behind this move is that it will help to provide more accurate counts of the incidence of CMFs.

One way to check the accuracy of the upward trend in the rates of CMFs is to use another comparable dataset to examine fatal maltreatment; however, there is no other source of information that measures and tracks CMFs in the U.S. Scholars in other countries, such as Germany and France, have also noted difficulty in gaining accurate counts of CMFs (Banaschak, Janssen, Schulte, & Rothschild, 2015; Tursz et al., 2010). A close approximation in the U.S. is the homicide rate among children. The Center for Health Statistics at the U.S. Centers for Disease Control and Prevention (CDC) collects the homicide rate among their vital statistics. The U.S. Federal Bureau of Investigation (FBI) also collects information about homicides through the Supplementary Homicide Reports. One can search for statistics about homicide on their respective websites and can limit the search by age of the victim in order to focus on children. The sources of homicide rates among children are approximations for CMFs only because homicide with child victims does not capture many deaths due to neglect (Bennett et al., 2006) and because homicide rates could include killings by nonfamily members, which would not be considered a

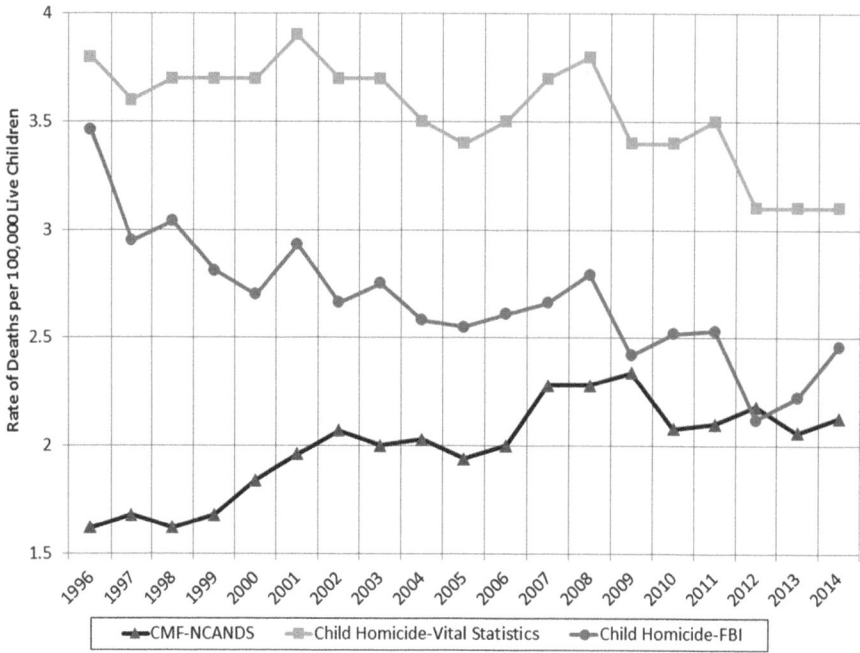

Figure 2.2 Comparison of Rate of Child Maltreatment Fatalities and Child Homicide in the United States 1996–2014 (*Sources: NCANDS data are for victims, ages 0–17. Vital Statistics rates from the Centers for Disease Control and Prevention are for child homicide victims, ages 0–4. FBI rates are for child homicide victims, ages 0–5.*)

maltreatment fatality. To help control for this latter complication, it is standard to only use rates among very young children since they are most likely to be killed by a family member (Bennett et al., 2006; Birken, Parkin, To, Wilkins, & Macarthur, 2009). The CMF and child homicide rates from the CDC and FBI rates are plotted in Figure 2.2.

Figure 2.2 shows that the two sources of information on homicides differ in their prevalence of the problem, but follow similar trends for this near 15-year period of time. Depending on which data source one uses, the homicide rate among children ages 0–4 or 5 has dropped between 13 and 27%. Meanwhile, Figure 2.1 shows that the rate of deaths by abuse or neglect has increased 44%. One potential conclusion is that the field has become better at recognizing when a child has been the victim of maltreatment—especially neglect—and that this may, in part, explain the rise in CMFs while the official homicide rate has declined. This will be further discussed in Chapter 9.

Changes in state law have also been known to affect the count of CMFs. Texas changed their child abuse and neglect statute so that if children are harmed as a result of their parents' drug use, it is considered maltreatment (Center for Public Policy Priorities, 2009). Another change in Texas law mandated that an autopsy be performed on all children under the age of 6 who die. It is speculated that this kind of legislative action (1) changes the way we conceptualize CMFs and (2) uncovers cases which might have previously been missed. In fact, in the 6 years before and 6 years after these legislative changes, there was a 68% increase in the number of CMFs in Texas, which was not paralleled in other states. This discussion brings us full circle back to the beginning of the chapter, which focused on definitions. This example from Texas provides clear evidence of how changes in definitions can yield changes in prevalence rates.

Even with local changes like this made all over the country, one cannot deny that even though national rates of non-fatal physical and sexual abuse have declined, rates of neglect have remained steady or increased. Between 1990 and the early 2000s the rates of physical abuse and sexual abuse declined 36% and 47%, respectively. Rates of neglect, however, did not have a clear linear progression and declined only 7% (Jones et al., 2006). These trends have continued into the current decade as well (Finkelhor & Jones, 2012). The next obvious question which follows is: how can rates of non-fatal abuse and neglect be declining while rates of CMF are increasing? Thus, one question is whether the CMF rate is the ultimate measure of abuse and neglect in the U.S. Given changes in legislative and agency policy and changes in practice by law enforcement and medical examiners, it is extremely challenging to track these rates over time. This is a question that officially remains unanswered. Nevertheless, by using data on non-fatal maltreatment and homicide among children and adults, one can come to some tentative conclusions, which will be further explored in Chapter 9 at the end of this book.

2.4 The Bottom Line

2.4.1 What We Know

This chapter provides an introduction to what we know and some of the controversies about fatal maltreatment. What we know is that even with changes and improvements in policy and practice, we undercount the number of children who die from abuse or neglect. If we use official statistics from recent years, somewhere between 1,500 and 1,700 children die each year in the U.S. It could be as high as 5,000, however (United States Advisory Board on Child Abuse and Neglect, 1995). Further, the way that we define a maltreatment-related death differs between states because how states define abuse and neglect differs. Additionally, a change in state or agency policy can drastically change the official incidence rate of CMFs, as happened in Texas. We also know that more children die from neglect than abuse, and specifically from supervisory neglect.

2.4.2 What Remains Unknown

What remains unknown about child abuse and neglect deaths in the U.S. is whether the rate of CMFs is increasing, decreasing, or staying the same. Making "progress" and changing policy and practice around CMFs is a double-edged sword: At the same time that we work on prevention, we work to better identify existing cases of CMFs, which means that there are a lot of moving parts; this makes getting accurate counts and a handle on trends over time difficult. A decline in the homicide rate among children age 0–5 may mean that prevention programs, such as public education initiatives around shaken baby syndrome/abusive head trauma may reduce the number of fatalities. At the same time, changes in how law enforcement and medical examiners practice may mean an increase in accurately identifying CMF cases that previously might have been classified as deaths by undetermined means or an accidental injury, for example. Further, advancements in emergency medicine mean that some children who would have died decades ago may be more likely to live today.

There has been movement among (CDRTs) to collect better data about the cases that they review (Cooper, 2008; Schnitzer, Covington, Wirtz, Verhoek-Oftedahl, & Palusci, 2008); see Chapter 5 for more information. Today there are protocols in place to gather standardized data and 35 states are voluntarily following these guidelines (Covington, 2011). (See Chapter 7 for more information.) There have also been calls to standardize the way that states define child abuse and neglect-related deaths so that we can accurately count CMFs to determine change over time (Chance, 2003); this is part of the mission of the federal commission which is intended to reduce CMFs in the U.S., the National Commission to Eliminate Child Abuse and Neglect Fatalities ("Protect Our Kids Act," 2012). Thus, if definitions and data collection techniques become standardized then it might be easier to gain a foothold on the incidence rates of CMFs.

As noted in Chapter 1, the phenomenon of fatal child maltreatment has been the focus of repeated efforts and resources. This has been a mixed blessing. On the one hand, it is fortunate that a social problem with a large impact, but low prevalence rate, can receive the level of resources that CMFs have received. At the same time, this input of attention from varied resources can have professionals, providers, decision-makers, and scholars running in different directions, all with the same intention—to lower the incidence of CMFs. The end result has been a high level of confusion, which stemmed from using different definitions, data collection, and practice techniques. There have been multiple efforts to reign in this confusion and to bring order to how we define, count, and address CMFs and this book documents and evaluates many of those efforts.

References

Adler, C., & Polk, K. (2001). *Child victims of homicide*. Cambridge, UK: Cambridge University Press.
Ahmad, O. B., Lopez, A. D., & Inoue, M. (2000). The decline in child mortality: A reappraisal. *Bulletin of the World Health Organization, 78*, 1175–1191.

References

Asser, S. M., & Swan, R. (1998). Child fatalities from religion-motivated medical neglect. *Pediatrics, 101*(4), 625.

Banaschak, S., Janssen, K., Schulte, B., & Rothschild, M. A. (2015). Rate of deaths due to child abuse and neglect in children 0–3 years of age in Germany. *International Journal of Legal Medicine, 129*(5), 1091–1096. doi:10.1007/s00414-015-1144-z.

Bennett, M. D., Jr., Hall, J., Frazier, L., Jr., Patel, N., Barker, L., & Shaw, K. (2006). Homicide of children aged 0–4 years, 2003–04: Results from the National Violent Death Reporting System. *Injury Prevention: Journal of the International Society for Child and Adolescent Injury Prevention, 12*(Suppl 2), ii39–ii43.

Berkowitz, C. D. (2003). Child neglect. In M. S. Peterson, M. Durfee, & K. Coulter (Eds.), *Child abuse and neglect: Guidelines for identification, assessment, and case management* (pp. 69–74). Volcano, CA: Volcano Press, Inc.

Birken, C. S., Parkin, P. C., To, T., Wilkins, R., & Macarthur, C. (2009). Neighborhood socioeconomic status and homicides among children in urban Canada. *Pediatrics, 123*(5), 815–819. doi:10.1542/peds.2008-0132.

Bureau of Justice Statistics. (2014). *Homicide*. Retrieved January 27, 2015, from http://www.bjs.gov/index.cfm?ty=tp&tid=311

Center for Public Policy Priorities. (2009). *Child abuse and neglect deaths in Texas*. Center for Public Policy Priorities.

Centers for Disease Control. (1999). Achievements in public health, 1900–1999: Healthier mothers and babies. *Morbidity and Mortality Weekly Report, 48*(38), 849–858.

Chance, T. C. (2003, July). *Our children are dying: Understanding and improving national maltreatment fatality data*. Paper presented at the 8th International family violence research conference, Portsmouth, NH.

Child and Family Services Improvement and Innovation Act, Pub. L. No. 112–34, H.R. 2883 Stat. (2011).

Child Maltreatment Research Listserv. (2009, August 25). [New bulletin: Updated Trends in Child Maltreatment, 2008].

Child Trends. (2012). Infant homicide. *Indicators on children and youth*. Retrieved October 17, 2013, from http://www.childtrends.org/?indicators=infant-homicide

Committee on Child Abuse and Neglect-American Academy of Pediatrics. (1994). Distinguishing sudden infant death syndrome from child abuse fatalities. *Pediatrics, 94*(1), 124–126.

Cooper, S. (2008). Child death review procedures are ready to be standardised. *Children & Young People Now, 3*–3.

Corsini, C. A., & Viazzo, P. P. (Eds.). (1993). *The decline of infant mortality in Europe, 1800–1950: Four national case studies*. Florence, Italy: UNICEF.

Covington, T. M. (2011). The US National Child Death Review Case Reporting System. *Injury Prevention, 17*, 34–37.

Dallas Police Department. (1994, August 31–September 2). Paper presented at the Crimes Against Children 1994: The 6th annual seminar presented by the Dallas Police Department & the Dallas Children's Advocacy Center, Dallas, Texas.

Davis, K. (2013, October 14). Court-martial begins Tuesday in Dyess child neglect case. *Military Times*. Retrieved from http://www.militarytimes.com/article/20131014/NEWS06/310140011/Court-martial-begins-Tuesday-Dyess-child-neglect-case

Douglas, E. M. (2012). Child welfare workers' training, knowledge, and practice concerns regarding child maltreatment fatalities: An exploratory, multi-state analysis. *Journal of Public Child Welfare, 6*(5), 659–677. doi:10.1080/15548732.2012.723975.

Ellement, J. R. (2013, October 11). Parents charged with manslaughter in 2011 death of baby in Marshfield. *Boston Globe*. Retrieved from http://www.bostonglobe.com/metro/2013/10/11/parents-marshfield-baby-girl-charged-with-homicide-poisoned-infant-with-opiates-formula-bottle-authorities-say/AvD5rEvXRaebHRG3cZUCkL/story.html

Ewigman, B., Kivlahan, C., & Land, G. (1993). The Missouri fatality study: Underreporting of maltreatment fatalities among children younger than five years of age, 1983 through 1986. *Pediatrics, 91*(2), 330.

Finkelhor, D., & Jones, L. M. (2012). *Have sexual abuse and physical abuse declined since the 1990s?* Durham, NH: Crimes Against Children Research Center, University of New Hampshire.

Finkelhor, D., Jones, L. M., & Shattuck, A. (2010). *Updated trends in child maltreatment, 2008*. Durham, NH: Crimes Against Children Research Center, University of New Hampshire.

Flaherty, E. G. M. H. L. (2013). Caregiver-fabricated illness in a child: A manifestation of child maltreatment. *Pediatrics, 132*(3), 590–597. doi:10.1542/peds.2013-2045.

Fox, J. A., & Zawitz, M. W. (2004). *Homicide trends in the United States: 2002 update*. Washington, DC: U.S. Department of Justice. Retrieved from http://www.bjs.gov/content/pub/pdf/htus02.pdf.

Garstang, J., & Sidebotham, P. (2008). Interagency training: Establishing a course in the management of unexpected childhood death. *Child Abuse Review, 17*(5), 352–361.

Gilchrist, J., Ballesteros, M. F., & Parker, E. M. (2012, April). Vital signs: Unintentional injury deaths among persons aged 0–19 years — United States, 2000–2009. *Morbidity and Mortality Weekly Report, 61*.

Harris, V. A., Rochette, L. M., & Smith, G. A. (2011). Pediatric injuries attributable to falls from windows in the United States in 1990–2008. *Pediatrics, 128*(3), 455–462. doi:10.1542/peds.2010-2687.

Herman-Giddens, M. E., Brown, G., Verbiest, S., Carlson, P. J., Hooten, E. G., Howell, E., et al. (1999). Underascertainment of child abuse mortality in the United States. *JAMA, 282*(5), 463–467.

Hymel, K. P., & Committee on Child Abuse and Neglect-American Academy of Pediatrics. (2006). Distinguishing sudden infant death syndrome from child abuse fatalities. *Pediatrics, 118*(1), 421–427.

Jones, L. M., & Finkelhor, D. (2003). Putting together evidence on declining trends in sexual abuse: A complex puzzle. *Child Abuse & Neglect, 27*(2), 133–135.

Jones, L. M., Finkelhor, D., & Halter, S. (2006). Child maltreatment trends in the 1990s: Why does neglect differ from sexual and physical abuse? *Child Abuse & Neglect, 11*(2), 107–120.

Kim, S. Y., Shapiro-Mendoza, C. K., Chu, S. Y., Camperlengo, L. T., & Anderson, R. N. (2012). Differentiating cause-of-death terminology for deaths coded as sudden infant death syndrome, accidental suffocation, and unknown cause: An investigation using US death certificates, 2003–2004. *Journal of Forensic Sciences, 57*(2), 364–369. doi:10.1111/j.1556-4029.2011.01937.x.

Klevens, J., & Leeb, R. T. (2010). Child maltreatment fatalities in children under 5: Findings from the National Violence Death Reporting System. *Child Abuse & Neglect: The International Journal, 34*(4), 262–266.

Lanning, K. V., & Walsh, B. (1996). Criminal investigation of suspected child abuse (From APSAC handbook on child maltreatment, pp. 246–270, 1996, John Briere, Lucy Berliner, et al. eds. – See NCJ-172299) *Criminal investigation of suspected child abuse (From APSAC handbook on child maltreatment, pp. 246–270, 1996, John Briere, Lucy Berliner, et al., eds. – See NCJ-172299)* (pp. 246–270). United States.

Levene, S., & Bacon, C. J. (2004). Sudden unexpected death and covert homicide in infancy. *Archives of Disease in Childhood, 89*(5), 443–447.

Liang, B. A., & Macfarlane, W. L. (1999, Summer). Murder by omission: Child abuse and the passive parent. *Harvard Journal on Legislation, 36*(2), 397–450.

Margolin, L. (1990). Fatal child neglect. *Child Welfare, 69*(4), 309–319.

Mash, C., Frazier, T., Nowacki, A., Worley, S., & Goldfarb, J. (2011). Development of a risk-stratification tool for medical child abuse in failure to thrive. *Pediatrics, 128*(6), e1467–e1473. doi:10.1542/peds.2011-1080.

McKee, G. R. (2006). *Why mothers kill: A forensic psychologist's casebook*. New York, NY: Oxford University Press.

McLaren, C., Null, J., & Quinn, J. (2005). Heat stress from enclosed vehicles: Moderate ambient temperatures cause significant temperature rise in enclosed vehicles. *Pediatrics, 116*(1), e109–e112. doi:10.1542/peds.2004-2368.

Meyer, C., Oberman, M., & Rone, M. (2001). *Mothers who kill their children: Understanding the acts of moms from Susan Smith to the "prom mom"*. New York, NY: New York University Press.

Miller, C. M., & Burch, A. D. S. (2013, August 20). Names of dead children invoked at hearing to reform DCF. *Miami Herald*. Retrieved from http://www.miamiherald.com/2013/08/20/3575635/names-of-dead-children-invoked.html#storylink=cpy

Murphy, S. L., Xu, J., & Kochanek, K. D. (2013). Deaths: Final data for 2010. *National Vital Statistics Report, 61*(3).

Murray, G. V. (2011, July 28). Judge acquits mother in death: 23-month-old fell from window. *Worcester Telegram & Gazette.* Retrieved from http://www.telegram.com/article/20110728/NEWS/107289464/0

National Conference of State Legislatures. (2011). Summary of the "Child and Family Services Improvement and Innovation Act" (S.1542/H.R. 2883). Retrieved December 21, 2013, from http://www.ncsl.org/research/human-services/summary-of-the-quotchild-and-family-services-imp.aspx

Palusci, V. J., & Covington, T. M. (2014). Child maltreatment deaths in the U.S. National Child Death Review Case Reporting System. *Child Abuse & Neglect, 38*(1), 25–36. doi:http://dx.doi.org/10.1016/j.chiabu.2013.08.014.

Pediatrics, C. o. C. A. a. N.-A. A. o. (2001). Distinguishing sudden infant death syndrome from child abuse fatalities. *Pediatrics, 107*(2), 437–441.

Pitcher, G. J., & Bowley, D. M. G. (2002). Infant rape in South Africa. *Lancet, 359*(9303), 274–275.

Protect Our Kids Act, Pub. L. No. 112–275 (2012).

Schnitzer, P. G., Covington, T. M., Wirtz, S. J., Verhoek-Oftedahl, W., & Palusci, V. J. (2008). Public health surveillance of fatal child maltreatment: Analysis of 3 state programs. *American Journal of Public Health, 98*(2), 296–303. doi:10.2105/ajph.2006.087783.

Schreier, H. A., & Libow, J. A. (1993). Munchausen syndrome by proxy: Diagnosis and prevalence. *American Journal of Orthopsychiatry, 63*(2), 318–321. doi:10.1037/h0079426.

Sethi, D., Bellis, M., Hughes, K., Gilbert, R., Mitis, F., & Galea, G. (2013). *European report on preventing child maltreatment.* Copenhagen, Denmark: World Health Organization Europe.

Shapiro-Mendoza, C. K., Kimball, M., Tomashek, K. M., Anderson, R. N., & Blanding, S. (2009). US infant mortality trends attributable to accidental suffocation and strangulation in bed from 1984 through 2004: Are rates increasing? *Pediatrics, 123*(2), 533–539. doi:10.1542/peds.2007-3746.

Soerdjbalie-Maikoe, V., Bilo, R. A. C., van den Akker, E., & Maes, A. (2010). Unnatural death due to child abuse – Forensic autopsies 1996–2009. *Nederlands Tijdschrift Voor Geneeskunde, 154*, A2285–A2285

Stevens, A. (2013, October 15). Paulding boy, 12, believed beaten to death. *Atlanta Constitution Journal.* Retrieved from http://www.ajc.com/news/news/paulding-boy-found-beaten-to-death/nbNZC/

Stirling, J., & Abuse, a. t. C. o. C., & Neglect. (2007). Beyond Munchausen syndrome by proxy: Identification and treatment of child abuse in a medical setting. *Pediatrics, 119*(5), 1026–1030. doi:10.1542/peds.2007-0563.

Swan, R. (1997). Children, medicine, religion and the law. *Advances in Pediatrics, 44*, 491–543.

Tsai, H.-L., Yang, L.-Y., Chin, T.-W., Chen, P.-H., Yen, H.-J., Liu, C.-S., … Chang, J.-W. (2012). Child abuse in medical setting presenting as gross hematuria: Diagnosis by DNA short tandem repeats. *Pediatrics, 130*(1), e224–e229. doi:10.1542/peds.2011-3271.

Tursz, A., Crost, M., Gerbouin-Rerolle, P., & Cook, J. M. (2010). Underascertainment of child abuse fatalities in France: Retrospective analysis of judicial data to assess underreporting of infant homicides in mortality statistics. *Child Abuse & Neglect: The International Journal, 34*(7), 534–544.

U.S. Bureau of Justice Statistics. (n.d.). *Homicide.* Retrieved October 17, 2013, from http://www.bjs.gov/index.cfm?ty=tp&tid=311

U.S. Children's Bureau. (2011). *Definitions of child abuse and neglect.* Washington, DC: Child Welfare Information Gateway. Retrieved from https://www.childwelfare.gov/systemwide/laws_policies/statutes/define.pdf

U.S. Department of Health & Human Services. (2011). *Child maltreatment 2010: Reports from the States to the National Child Abuse and Neglect Data Systems – National statistics on child abuse and neglect.* Washington, DC: Administration for Children & Families, U.S. Department of Health & Human Services.

U.S. Department of Health & Human Services. (2012). *Child maltreatment 2011: Reports from the States to the National Child Abuse and Neglect Data Systems – National statistics on child abuse and neglect*. Washington, DC: Administration for Children & Families, U.S. Department of Health & Human Services.

U.S. Department of Health & Human Services. (2013). *Child maltreatment 2012: Reports from the States to the National Child Abuse and Neglect Data Systems – National statistics on child abuse and neglect*. Washington, DC: Administration for Children & Families, U.S. Department of Health & Human Services.

U.S. Department of Health & Human Services. (2015). *Child maltreatment 2013: Reports from the States to the National Child Abuse and Neglect Data Systems – National statistics on child abuse and neglect*. Washington, DC: Administration for Children & Families, U.S. Department of Health & Human Services.

UNICEF. (2003). *A league table of child maltreatment deaths in rich countries*. Innocent report card, issue no. 5 September 2003. Retrieved October 26, 2003, from http://www.unicef-icdc.org/publications/

United Nations Children's Fund. (2015). *Levels & trends in child mortality*. New York, NY: United Nations Children's Fund.

United States Advisory Board on Child Abuse and Neglect. (1995). *A nation's shame: Fatal child abuse and neglect in the United States*.

Young, M., & Hyden, P. W. (2003). Child abuse by burning. In M. S. Peterson, M. Durfee, & K. Coulter (Eds.), *Child abuse and neglect: Guidelines for identification, assessment, and case management* (pp. 41–47). Volcano, CA: Volcano Press, Inc.

Chapter 3
Risk Factors for Fatal Maltreatment Victimization and Perpetration

The media is filled with heart-breaking stories of children of all ages who die from abuse and neglect. This selection of stories about child fatalities told in the media paints a picture which is not necessarily representative of all cases of fatal maltreatment and can mislead readers, including the public and helping professionals, about what places a child at-risk for fatality. This chapter will begin by identifying known and accepted risk factors that increase the probability that a child will become the victim of a maltreatment fatality. Some of these include a child's age and gender, parent/perpetrator age, parent mental health concerns, and social/environmental conditions in the home. The second portion of the chapter will focus on the areas of controversy concerning risk factors for child maltreatment fatalities (CMFs), including parent/perpetrator gender, race of victim/parent/perpetrator, child behavioral health, and the parent-child relationship. These controversies are fueled by a variety of sources, including the media and historically uninformed assumptions about the "goodness" and limits of parents' actions toward their children. The chapter will end by covering some risk factors which have been inadequately explored which prevent professionals from more accurately identifying children who are at risk for a maltreatment death. For the sake of remaining true to the book's form, I highlight the areas of controversy here:

- Women are more likely to be responsible for children's deaths due to maltreatment than men.
- African American/Black children are more likely to be victims of CMFs than children in other race/ethnic groups.
- About one-third to one-half of children who die from maltreatment are known to child protective services before the child's death.
- Children who die from maltreatment are more likely to be described as "difficult," but their parents may have inadequate knowledge of child development.

3.1 Commonly Accepted Risk Factors

3.1.1 Child Age

What victims of fatal maltreatment have most in common is their age. The strongest risk factor for becoming a victim of a CMF is being a young child—a very young child. The research overwhelmingly finds that children under the age of 1, are at the greatest risk of being killed or dying from maltreatment; in fact, the risk for homicide is 10 times greater on the first day of life than at any other time (Paulozzi, 2002). There is no disagreement about this; it is a well-established fact in the child welfare and health professions. Text box 3.1 describes a typical scenario.

Text Box 3.1
Michael Sanchez, Jr., 9 months old, was found dead in his crib in Texas. He was wrapped in wet blankets; he was cold, stiff, and rigor mortis had started to set in. Michael's family had a long history of involvement with child protective services and often had law enforcement call to his home (Casady, 2013).

The annual *Child Maltreatment* report published by the U.S. Department of Health & Human Services, and that I discussed in Chapter 2, shows that most of the children who die from abuse or neglect are under the age of 4. Between 2010 and 2014, 45.0% of CMF victims were under 1 year old and 79.4% were under 4 years old (U.S. Department of Health & Human Services, 2011–2015). These findings are consistent with the literature using other national and state sources of information. The U.S. National Child Death Review Case Reporting System found that of maltreatment-related cases reviewed at the state-level between 2005 and 2009, about one-half involved infant victims (Palusci & Covington, 2014). The National Violence Death Reporting System which is maintained by the U.S. Centers for Disease Control and Prevention found that infants make up just over half of deaths in their databases, but make up two-thirds of neglect-related deaths (Klevens & Leeb, 2010). Child age is not a newly known risk factor for CMF; a national study of parent-perpetrated child homicides using the Uniform Crime Reports between 1976 and 1985 (which does not always include cases of neglect, see Chapter 2 for more information), found that almost 40% of victims were killed before they reached their first birthday; 9% died in the first week of life. Overall, 78% of the victims were under the age of 5 (Kunz & Bahr, 1996). State-level data tells a similar story with regard to a young childhood being a risk factor for fatal maltreatment (Anderson, Ambrosino, Valentine, & Lauderdale, 1983; Beveridge, 1994).

3.1.2 Child Gender

Most studies have found a slightly higher rate of male than female victimization; between 2010 and 2014, 58.6% of victims of abuse and neglect-related deaths in the U.S. were male (U.S. Department of Health & Human Services, 2011–2015). Two large-scale national data collection systems also find that males are more likely to die than females: U.S. National Child Death Review Case Reporting System—56% (Palusci & Covington, 2014) and the National Violence Death Reporting System—59% (Klevens & Leeb, 2010). Between 1976 and 1985, 55% of child homicide victims in the U.S. who were killed by their parents were male (Kunz & Bahr, 1996). Similar findings have been reported using state-level data as well (Anderson et al., 1983; Beveridge, 1994; Lucas et al., 2002). An older study which used data from Iowa, found that in the 1980s, 71% of victims of fatal neglect were male (Margolin, 1990). Research on fatal maltreatment in Oklahoma from 1986 to 2006 compared fatal neglect with fatal abuse and found that there was no statistical gender difference between victims of fatal abuse, even though victims of fatal neglect were more likely to be male (Damashek, Nelson, & Bonner, 2013; Welch & Bonner, 2013). The slightly higher rate of CMFs among male children may be explained by the fact that the birth rate is slightly higher for males than for females (Martin et al., 2012) and that most victims die early in life.

3.1.3 Parent/Perpetrator Age

Most perpetrators are in young adulthood, which is not surprising given the age of the victims and the age at which most people are parents to young children. Kunz and Bahr (1996) found that roughly 70% of perpetrators are under the age of 30. In a study of fatally abandoned newborn infants, Herman-Giddens, Smith, Mittal, Carlson and Butts (2003) also found that 77% of the mothers were less than 30. Other studies have estimated that the majority of perpetrators are in their 20s, with a minority in their teens or 30s (Damashek et al., 2013; Levine, Freeman, & Compaan, 1994). My own analysis of the National Child Abuse and Neglect Data System (NCANDS) data showed that parents of fatally maltreated children were 29.5 years of age, and that they were slightly younger than parents of non-fatally maltreated children (Douglas & Mohn, 2014).

3.1.4 Socioeconomic Status

With some exceptions (Chance & Scannapieco, 2002), research finds that poverty, financial hardship, receipt of need-based services, and lower levels of education and income are risk factors for fatal maltreatment (Meyer, Oberman, & Rone, 2001; Oberman & Meyer, 2008). In the comparative study that I completed with a colleague using NCANDS, we found that families which experienced a CMF were more likely to have financial problems (Douglas & Mohn, 2014); a descriptive study of CMFs from Texas found that most victims came from families working "blue collar" jobs (Anderson et al., 1983). A recent study from the U.S. National Child Death Review Case Reporting System found that 25% of CMF victims were receiving Medicaid at the time of their death. Similarly, another study found that children whose mothers do not have a high school education are at an increased risk of 1.7% for fatal maltreatment when compared to children who died of natural causes (Stiffman, Schnitzer, Adam, Kruse, & Ewigman, 2002). Much of this research is descriptive in nature or only considers differences between fatal and non-fatal victims one characteristic at a time, as opposed to a constellation of factors at once. Nevertheless, the evidence indicates that children living in families experiencing financial difficulties or with low levels of education are at a higher risk for a maltreatment fatality.

3.1.5 Household Risk Factors

Most children who die from maltreatment live with their biological parents. The terminology on this aspect of children's lives has changed over time: some studies report on mother's marital status; others report on the adults with whom the children lived and the relationships of those individuals to the children. At a minimum, we know that children who die from maltreatment most commonly lived with their mothers (Douglas & Mohn, 2014; Margolin, 1990; Palusci & Covington, 2014; Sinal et al., 2000). In addition, one-third to one-half of children also lived with their fathers. Data from NCANDS tells us that 50% of CMF victims lived with both of their parents when they died. Meanwhile, data from the multi-state U.S. National Child Death Review Case Reporting System shows that the majority of children lived with unmarried mothers (Palusci & Covington, 2014). State-level data provides similar estimates: in Oklahoma, 45% of children lived with their married parents, although 69% of children lived with both of their parents, married or not (Damashek et al., 2013); estimates show that in Missouri, among children who died from CMF, 41–56% of children lived with both of their parents (Schnitzer & Ewigman, 2008; Stiffman et al., 2002); finally, among CMF victims in Kansas, 38% lived with a married mother (Kajese et al., 2011). When victims did not live with both parents, they were most likely to live with their mothers alone (Douglas & Mohn, 2014; Palusci & Covington, 2014).

Children are more at-risk of suffering a maltreatment fatality in homes that have recently experienced a major life event, such as moving, unemployment, or the birth of a child (Lucas et al., 2002). One study found that among families experiencing a CMF, 26% had an unemployed parent and 40% had moved within the last year; overall, families had a high degree of mobility (Anderson et al., 1983), which is consistent with other descriptive research on fatal maltreatment (Douglas, 2013). In fact, with some exception (Palusci & Covington, 2014), housing and household composition appear to be important risk factors for CMFs. As compared with children who died of natural causes, children who live with non-family members are ten times more likely to become CMF victims than children who live with two birth parents (Stiffman et al., 2002). Other research has confirmed that children who become CMF victims have more people residing in their homes and are likely to have had a recent change in household composition (Chance & Scannapieco, 2002).

3.2 Areas of Controversy

3.2.1 *Perpetrator Characteristics*

Children are actively or passively killed by their caregivers or people they know. Between 2010 and 2014, over three-quarters (78.7%) of CMFs were perpetrated by a parent acting alone or in combination with another person (U.S. Department of Health & Human Services, 2011–2015). An additional 3.1% of perpetrators are the partners of parents and may perform caregiving responsibilities; 0.4% are foster parents. In addition to this, 3.7% of perpetrators are relatives and 1.8% are daycare providers (U.S. Department of Health & Human Services, 2012). Thus, children are overwhelmingly killed by the adults in their lives who are charged with the responsibility of caring for and protecting them. Other research has shown that when the perpetrator is not the biological parent, it is most commonly the parent's partner—a step-father or mother's boyfriend (Levine et al., 1994; Palusci & Covington, 2014).

Women are most likely to perpetrate or be responsible for the deaths of children. Between 2010 and 2014, 39.3% of CMFs were committed by mothers or mothers and another individual, 17.1% were committed by fathers or fathers and another individual and 22.3% were committed by mothers and fathers together (U.S. Department of Health & Human Services, 2011–2015), which means that mothers were involved 61.6% of the time and fathers were involved in CMFs 39.4% of the time. Similar rates were found in a recent study of cases examined by child death review teams in 23 states. Among all maltreatment deaths, the perpetrator was female 52% of the time; among instances where neglect was present, the perpetrator was female 85% of the time; among instances where physical abuse was present, the perpetrator was female 26% of the time (Palusci & Covington, 2014). Similar figures were found among the U.S. Uniform Crime Reports of parent-to-child homicides, with 52.5% of perpetrators being mothers (Kunz & Bahr, 1996); an older study of CMFs in Iowa found that mothers were responsible for CMF deaths 41% of the time and specifically, for neglect deaths 53% of the time (Margolin, 1990). Presumably, mothers are more often the perpetrators because mothers spend more time with children (Manlove & Vernon-Feagans, 2002; Wood & Repetti, 2004). Finally, most perpetrators are in early adulthood (Chance & Scannapieco, 2002; Herman-Giddens et al., 2003; Kunz & Bahr, 1996; Meyer et al., 2001; Yampolskaya, Greenbaum, & Berson, 2009).

The information that I have presented thus far about perpetrators is not challenged by scholars of maltreatment and family violence, but there is some evidence that this is less well known by child welfare professionals and perhaps the general public. A study that I conducted in 2010–2011 of over 450 child welfare workers across the country showed that only 20% knew that mothers were most often responsible for children's deaths and only 38% appropriately identified family members as most often being responsible for children's deaths (Douglas, 2012). Further, when I present this information at conferences and trainings, I am often questioned about the legitimacy of the information and told that the NCANDS data that I am presenting does not match what happens in "their" state. I know of no other research that investigates the knowledge of professionals or the general public about characteristics of perpetrators of CMFs, but the results of this one study and my own individual experiences suggest that there is a significant gap in knowledge about risk factors for perpetration of a CMF.

3.2.2 Prior Involvement with Child Welfare/Social Services

Children who die are often known to child welfare or social services—something which lights a fire under both the public, advocates, and state decision-makers (Miller & Burch, 2013b). In fact, having been the subject of a report to a child maltreatment hotline considerably raises one's risk of becoming a CMF victim (Jonson-Reid, Chance, & Drake, 2007; Sabotta & Davis, 1992). Data from the National Child Death Review Case Reporting System shows that 33% of CMF victims were previously known to child protective services (Palusci & Covington, 2014). Of children who died from maltreatment in Oklahoma from 1986 to 2006, 32% of the victims had been the subject of a child abuse or neglect report, but 49% of the victims' families had been a subject of a report for either the deceased child or another family member. This was more common among children who died of neglect (Damashek et al., 2013). Further, among neglect-related deaths, 49% had current involvement with human services (i.e., food stamps) and 12% had been in contact with child protective services within 3 months prior to their death (Welch & Bonner, 2013). Similarly, 30% of children in Missouri who died of a maltreatment-related fatality had been in contact with child welfare services prior to their death (Schnitzer & Ewigman, 2008) and one third (34.1%) of victims of child abuse deaths in Kansas from 1994 to 2007 were known, or their families were known, to child protective services prior to their death (Kajese et al., 2011). Older research shows that among Texas children who died from abuse or neglect in the 1970s, about one-quarter were known to child welfare services prior to their death (Anderson et al., 1983). In sum, about one-third to one-half of children who die from maltreatment are known to child protective services.

Sometimes children have been in foster care and have been reunited with their families before they die. The annual *Child Maltreatment* reports show that between 2010 and 2014, 11% of children who died came from families that had received family preservation services in the past 5 years and just under 2% had been reunified with their families in the past 5 years after an out of home placement (U.S. Department of Health & Human Services, 2011–2015). Information from the U.S. National Death Review Case Reporting System shows that 9% of children who died from maltreatment had formerly been in foster care (Palusci & Covington, 2014). At the same time, one study showed that having been in an out-of-home placement decreased risk CMFs (Chance & Scannapieco, 2002). Finally, some children also die when they are in out-of-home care, but it is a small percent; between 2010 and 2014 less than 1% of perpetrators were foster parents or residential/group home staff (U.S. Department of Health & Human Services, 2011–2015).

The public, media, and legislatures often express outrage when a child whose family is working with child protective services dies from maltreatment (Carrier, 2002; Davis, 1987). The flip side of this, however, is that if 30–50% of children who become victims of CMF are known to child protective services, that means that 30–70% of CMF victims are unknown to protective agencies. There is no research that focuses on the potential differences between children who have been reported to child protective services and become CMF victims and children who were never reported, but also become CMF victims. Information from such a study could help to identify additional children who are at-risk and in the community.

3.2.3 Race and Ethnicity of Victims and Perpetrators

There are racial and ethnic disparities among victims of CMFs. This disparity has the most negative impact on Black/African Americans and American Indians because they are over-represented among CMF victims (Herman-Giddens et al., 2003; Kunz & Bahr, 1996; U.S. Department of Health & Human Services, 2015). For example, as Table 3.1 shows, on average between 2010 and 2014, almost 16% of the child population in the United States was Black/African American. Yet, 25% of CMFs victims nationwide were Black/African American, which means that among CMF victims, Black children are represented at almost twice their presence in the

Table 3.1 Child Population and CMF Victimization by Race and Ethnicity[a]

Race/Ethnicity	Percent of the Child Population 2010–2014	Percent of CMF Victims 2010–2014
African American	15.69	25.11
American Indian/Alaska Native	0.91	1.09
Asian	3.59	0.85
Hispanic/Latino	20.82	13.15
Pacific Islander	0.15	0.18
Unknown	–	6.46
White/Caucasian	55.34	40.94

[a]Source: U.S. Department of Health & Human Services (2011–2015). Annual *Child Maltreatment* reports

population at large, These findings regarding race were confirmed by other recent national databases including data from the U.S. National Child Death Review Case Reporting System (Palusci & Covington, 2014) and the National Violence Death Reporting System (Klevens & Leeb, 2010). With some exceptions (Jason & Andereck, 1983; Sinal et al., 2000), these findings have paralleled research at the state level. A review of published and unpublished literature on child fatalities found that African American children were represented at three times their rate as in the general population (Levine et al., 1994). A recent study on fatal neglect in Oklahoma also found that CMF victims were three times more likely to be Black as compared to their presence in the population. (Welch & Bonner, 2013). A high percentage of African American CMF victims have also been confirmed in Missouri (Stiffman et al., 2002) and North Carolina (Herman-Giddens et al., 2003).

American Indian children were also slightly over-represented as CMF victims, as compared to their presence in the child population. On average, they comprise 1% of victims, which slightly over-represents their presence in the general population (U.S. Department of Health & Human Services, 2011–2015). This over-representation has been noted at the state level, too. The study of victims of fatal neglect in Oklahoma noted that 13% of the victims were American Indian, even though American Indians comprise only 9% of the state's population (Welch & Bonner, 2013).

According to the national statistics reported in Table 3.1, Hispanic or Latino children are slightly underrepresented among CMF victims. Of course, this can vary significantly by region. For example, one older study in Texas found that 24% of the CMF victims in Texas were Mexican-American (Anderson et al., 1983)—a finding that is likely important for southwestern states, but potentially less helpful for other regions, such as New England—when considering prevention efforts, because of less racial diversity in that region. Asian children, as well as White/Caucasian children are also underrepresented among fatal victims of abuse and neglect.

These findings with regard to race and ethnicity are not unique to fatal maltreatment. Similar statistics exist with regard to non-fatal child maltreatment as well (Knott & Donovan, 2010) and have been explained by two overriding perspectives: (1) social/economic stress and (2) disproportionality. Racism and discrimination are what, in part, provide support for the social/economic stress theory of child maltreatment, which was largely developed in the 1970s (Gelles, 1973, 1996). This perspective, also called the "risk model" (Drake et al., 2011), suggests that families which endure particular social/economic stressors, such as poverty, racism, low levels of education, housing difficulties, domestic violence, and so forth, are at an increased risk for maltreatment (Delsordo & Leavitt, 1974; Gelles, 1978; Gelles & Harrop, 1991; Mapp, 2006; Stith et al., 2009; Whipple, 1999; World Health Organization, 2001). The social/economic stress model is the basis for the modern-day child welfare and social service system. Families are given supportive services to alleviate their stress and, in theory, the risk for maltreatment declines (Delsordo & Leavitt, 1974; Gelles, 1973). According to this perspective, Black/African American and American Indian children are subjected to more maltreatment because racism creates a social environment filled with more adversity. Even though this perspective is now 40 years old, recent research shows support for this model (Drake et al., 2011).

A second perspective is that African American or American Indian children, whose ancestors endured long-term racism and hardship, continue to be the subjects of discrimination which leads to more reports and determinations of child maltreatment. According to this perspective, minority children are not abused any more than majority children, but they are more likely to be reported to the authorities or more likely to be the subject of a "false positive," which means to identify a problem when, in fact, none exists (Crofoot & Harris, 2012; Drake et al., 2011; Foster, 2012; Sinha, Trocmé, Fallon, & MacLaurin, 2013). Recent research shows support for this perspective (Foster, 2012), too; sometimes called the "bias theory" (Drake et al., 2011), but commonly termed "disproportionality." This problem is the focus of many interventions within the child welfare workforce today (Anyon, 2011; Clark, Buchanan, & Legters, 2008; Cross, 2008; Dettlaff & Rycraft, 2008; Knott & Giwa, 2012).

Some have suggested that CMFs might be the ultimate measure of child abuse and neglect in our nation. If more children from one population die from maltreatment, then maltreatment must be highest among that group of individuals (Child Maltreatment Research Listserv, 2009). This perspective is consistent with the social/economic stress theory. The disproportionality perspective reveals another side of the coin: more African American or American Indian child deaths may be incorrectly classified as due to maltreatment than their counterparts in other racial/ethnic groups. In this instance, medical examiners or coroners would (presumably) unintentionally be more likely to consider abuse or neglect when they are determining the death of a child, which could either lead to an accurate or an inaccurate diagnosis of maltreatment—a true positive or a false positive, respectively. The starting point is as important as the end result in this situation. If bias plays a role from the start there will be more determinations of CMF for African American and American Indian children than children from other ethnic groups. The child welfare profession has not resolved the controversy over what "causes" higher incidences of maltreatment among some racial groups; it is likely a multifaceted problem. Whatever the cause, it is reflected among victims of fatal and non-fatal maltreatment alike.

3.2.4 Child Behavior, Knowledge of Child Development, and the Parent-Child Relationship

> **Text Box 3.2**
> Aliyah Marie Branum was 2 years old when she was killed by her mother in the state of Florida in 2013. Aliyah's medical, physical, nutritional, and emotional needs were routinely neglected by her mother. She was also the subject of extraordinarily hard discipline techniques and physical abuse. Her mother suggested that she had trouble managing her daughter's emotions and behaviors. It was reported that when she was unable to quiet Aliyah she would put a blanket over Aliyah's mouth and hit her legs hard enough to leave welts. Her mother also reported that Aliyah would not listen and as a result, became
>
> (continued)

Text Box 3.2 (continued)
increasingly angry with her daughter. On the day of her death, her mother indicated that she could no longer tolerate Aliyah's cries, so she covered her daughter's mouth with her hand, shook her, and eventually threw her against a wall. Police report that upon her death, her face was puffy, one of her eyes was swollen shut, her skull was cracked and she bled from her nose and ears. She had injuries to her forehead, cheeks, lips, head, shoulders, pelvic area and back (Miller & Burch, 2013a).

3.2.4.1 Child Behavior and the Parent-Child Relationships

The story about the death of Aliyah Marie Branum, which is described in Text Box 3.2, is fairly common, or portions of it are common throughout different stories on maltreatment. It describes a mother whose parenting was out of control, but also a mother who found her child difficult to manage. It is the approach that the field takes to children's behavior that places this risk factor in the section on controversies. Research has shown that having a behavior problem places a child at risk for fatality, but it is unclear if behavioral problems can explain all of this risk or if parent knowledge of child development may play an important role, too.

Child behavior, or how a parent perceives his or her child to behave, has been examined by only a handful of studies; the results suggest that it may be an important element in understanding and identifying risk factors for fatal maltreatment. I surveyed child welfare workers in the U.S. who experienced a CMF on their caseload. I asked workers to describe the child who died and the child's family. Over one-third of workers indicated that the parents of the children who died saw their children as "difficult or ill behaved" (Douglas, 2013). Three studies that have been conducted on fatal and non-fatal child maltreatment among families involved with the child welfare system and that also considered child behavior problems. The first, a bivariate study—where only two variables are compared at a time—of fatal versus non-fatal maltreatment and child/family characteristics, found that children who were described as having provoking behaviors were 8.4 times more likely to die from abuse or neglect than children who did not have provoking behaviors (Chance & Scannapieco, 2002). The sample size for this study was small with only a total of 70 cases and the findings are inconsistent with a set of bivariate analyses that a colleague and I carried out with the NCANDS data (Douglas & Mohn, 2014). As a reminder to readers, NCANDS data is information that each state's child welfare system collects about their annual activities; it is compiled at the national level by the U.S. Administration on Children and Families; (see Chapter 2 for more information). We used the NCANDS data and restricted the sample to only cases where the child was determined to be a victim of maltreatment prior to the child's death. In other words, we did not include cases where a report to child protective services was screened out or where an investigation determined that no maltreatment was present. We found that children who had behavioral problems were *less* likely to die from maltreatment. Specifically, only 0.6% of children who were victims of fatal maltreatment were identified as having a behavioral problem, as compared to 3.6% of children who were victims of non-fatal maltreatment.

The third comparative study of fatal and non-fatal maltreatment focused on 540 "less-severe" child welfare cases within the Texas child protective system; this data was drawn from administrative case files from 1992 to 1996 and included 111 CMFs; the remainder of the sample was a comparison group. Among these seemingly lower risk cases, the researchers found that having a child behavior problem alone actually reduced risk of fatality. The authors suggest that risk factors which were deemed more "actionable" likely led to interventions on the part of child welfare professionals and thus, reduced the risk for fatality. At the same time, however, the combination of both a child behavior problem and parental stress increased the risk for fatality by a factor of 7. It is not clear why a child behavior problem in combination with parent stress would have been less "actionable." Whatever the case, the combination of child behavior and parent stress was a lethal combination for the children in that state sample.

One scholar developed a matrix of risk factors for maternal filicide, where infant temperament is one of the four elements listed under "situational factors" that can place a child at-risk for a fatal outcome (McKee, 2006). One example of this is a small study of 23 middle-class, well-educated mothers who had infants with colic; the researchers examined how mothers responded to their children's difficult temperament (Levitzky & Cooper, 2000). Sixteen of the mothers reported having fantasies about actively hurting or abandoning their infants, or of their children accidentally getting hurt as a result of the parents' every day actions; six of the mothers reported fantasizing about infanticide. Similarly, in a study of 32 children who died from physical abuse, 58% of the perpetrators—who were primarily male—disclosed that "prolonged crying" was the impetus for the fatal abuse (Brewster et al., 1998).

Text Box 3.3
Logan Marr was 5 years old and living in the state in Maine when she died in foster care in 2001. Her story was the subject of a *Frontline* documentary on PBS and showed that Logan was prone to rages. Her foster mother, a former child welfare worker, did not know how to handle Logan's temper tantrums. Her final outburst ended with her foster mother placing her in a high chair in their basement and wrapping her head and body in 40 feet of duct tape. Logan suffocated to death (Dretzin, Goodman, & Soenens, 2003).

Related to this, there is a strong body of research which shows that children with behavioral problems can elicit a harsher style of discipline from their parents and are at an increased risk for maltreatment (Blackson, Tarter, & Maezzich, 1996; Engfer & Schneewind, 1982; Sherrod, Altemeier, O'Connor, & Vietze, 1984; Tourigny, 2006), such as described in Text Box 3.3. Research in the 1970s showed that toddlers who were maltreated were more likely to physically assault their caregivers and to retreat from their caregivers' friendly overtures (George & Main, 1979). Thus, it is unclear whether parents perceive their children to be more difficult and thus, respond with more harsh disciplinary actions or if parents who use harsh disciplinary actions shape their children to have more behavioral problems. More recent publications concerning mothers who kill their children have addressed disciplinary techniques that "got out of control," but there has been little discussion around children's behavior as a contributing factor or explanatory reason (Meyer et al., 2001; O'Malley, 2004; Oberman & Meyer, 2008). Children's behavior, or how parents and caretakers perceive children's behavior appears to play an important role as a predictor of CMFs. In truth, however, this area of research is fraught with inconsistencies and we still have much to learn.

3.2.4.2 Parent Knowledge of Child Development and the Parent-Child Relationship

There is research which suggests that parent knowledge of child development may mask what parents and others call "child behavior problems." The most poignant examples of this come from a study that was conducted in the 1980s—a study of nine women who were incarcerated for killing or contributing to their children's deaths (Korbin, 1987). The women noted their children's behavioral problems as being linked to the killings, which included prolonged crying, talking back to the parents, toileting accidents, refusing to eat, or asking to return to a foster home. The women also noted instances of when children showed a lack of respect for their parents' hard work, such as when an infant "failed" to respect his mother's busy schedule by "squirming" too much during bath-time. In another instance the mother described her husband's fatal rage as being inspired by their infant's "unwillingness" to eat after his father worked all night to provide enough money for the family. In these situations, parents either lost control and lashed out at their children or engaged in physical discipline which got out of hand. These findings are similar to other research which was conducted on women who were incarcerated for the deaths of their children (Oberman & Meyer, 2008). This research raises the issue of whether the key component is a child's difficult behavior or whether parents have inappropriate expectations for their children and lack knowledge around normal child development.

There has been very little work completed in this area, however. In my descriptive study of child welfare workers who experienced the death of a child on their caseload, 65% of workers stated that in situations where children died, parents had age-inappropriate expectations of their children (Douglas, 2013). This finding parallels a small British study of male caregivers who violently killed young children; many of the men had unreasonable expectations of the children, treated them like small adults, or stated that they didn't know what to expect from a child (Cavanagh, Dobash, & Dobash, 2007). The Texas study which compared children in the child welfare system who died versus who lived, and which only considered one characteristic at a time, found that children were more likely to die when parents had "unrealistic expectations" of them (Chance & Scannapieco, 2002). Finally, the larger Texas comparative study, which examined multiple characteristics at once, found that when a parent had low levels of "parenting knowledge" children's risk for either abuse or neglect-related deaths more than doubled; when just abuse-related deaths were considered, children who were cared for by parents who had low levels of knowledge were eight times more likely to die from abuse than children whose parents had higher levels of knowledge. This same study also found that children who have parents with low levels of caring and attachment are at an increased risk for fatality, which is another important piece of information when considering the parent-child relationship (Graham, Stepura, Baumann, & Kern, 2010). It is unclear whether being a child with a difficult temperament or being a parent with low knowledge of child development—or both—places a child at risk for death. Thus far, there is evidence to say that both are risk factors and are potential entry points for intervention.

3.3 Unconfirmed Research

Most of the research on fatal child maltreatment focuses on the demographic information of victims, perpetrators, and their living situations: age, gender, race and ethnicity, socioeconomic status of the family, individuals living in the home and their relationships to one another, employment status and the like. This kind of information is easiest to obtain; it is available through the records of medical examiners, law enforcement, courts, health providers, and child welfare services. Information which goes beyond this, such as family social isolation, partner violence in the home, the parent-child relationship, or discipline techniques, can be difficult to obtain, especially if the family was not receiving or was not compliant with social services and health care.

3.3.1 Parent Mental Health

Several studies have found parental mental illness to be present in cases where children die from maltreatment. In a study that I conducted where child welfare workers described the characteristics of families that had a child die from maltreatment, over half of the parents had a problem with mental illness (Douglas, 2013). In other descriptive studies, researchers have noted parental mental health problems as a contributing factor in cases of CMFs (Brewster et al., 1998; Fein, 1979; Korbin, 1987; Margolin, 1990), especially among older victims (Lucas et al., 2002). A comparative study of fatal and non-fatal maltreatment in Florida found that mothers with behavioral health problems were more likely to fatally assault their children than mothers without such problems (Yampolskaya et al., 2009). At the same time, a Texas-based study which compared fatal and non-fatal child maltreatment found that parental mental health and substance abuse did not distinguish between fatal and non-fatal maltreatment (Chance & Scannapieco, 2002). Similarly, when a colleague and I compared fatal and non-fatal maltreatment using the NCANDS data, we did not find that parental emotional status differentiated between fatal and non-fatal victims (Douglas & Mohn, 2014).

3.3.2 Social Isolation

Social isolation has been noted as a risk factor for non-fatal maltreatment (Berlin, Appleyard, & Dodge, 2011; Hamilton, 1989), but has not been strongly linked to fatal maltreatment. In the study that I conducted of child welfare workers who lost a child client to fatality, only 14% described the families as having been socially isolated before the fatality. A comparative study of fatal and non-fatal maltreatment found that social isolation was not a distinguishing feature of CMFs (Chance & Scannapieco, 2002). Finally, a descriptive study of incarcerated women who were involved in killing their children found that these mothers had robust sources of social support (Korbin, 1998); in one other study of incarcerated women, however, the women themselves identified their isolation from others a determining factor in their children's demise (Oberman & Meyer, 2008).

3.3.3 Domestic Violence

Domestic violence is another area where there are mixed results about how it is potentially related to risk for a CMF. One study found that having a caretaker who was aggressive, but not necessarily within an intimate relationship, increased risk for fatal maltreatment among families already working with child welfare services (Graham et al., 2010). Similarly, another study of fatal and non-fatal maltreatment found that the presence of domestic violence among families involved with the child welfare system increased risk for fatality (Yampolskaya et al., 2009); and, a study of women who were incarcerated for their children's deaths found that women described relationships filled with domestic violence (Oberman & Meyer, 2008). But, not all research has agreed with these findings. Two studies that compared fatal and non-fatal victims of maltreatment found the presence of domestic violence did not increase risk for fatality (Chance & Scannapieco, 2002; Douglas & Mohn, 2014). This, too, is an area which deserves more attention in future research.

3.3.4 Child Disability Status

A small body of research has examined other characteristics of victims of CMFs. One descriptive study found that of children who died of maltreatment deaths, 17% had a disability or chronic illness (Palusci & Covington, 2014). Two studies which compared fatal and non-fatal outcomes did not find a statistically significant difference between victims with regard to disability status, cognitive impairments, or health concerns/medical conditions (Chance & Scannapieco, 2002; Douglas & Mohn, 2014). That said, a recent study that I conducted with the NCANDS data file shows that children who are known to the child welfare system and who have a physical disability or a medical condition are more at risk of dying from neglect (Douglas, 2016).

3.4 The Bottom Line

3.4.1 What We Know

The field is very clear about what we know with regard to risk factors for CMF.

- Children tend to be very young; the vast majority is under the age of 4 and close to half are under the age of 1.
- We also know that males are victimized slightly more frequently than females. Sometimes this difference is large enough to have statistical significance, other times it is not.
- The literature is very clear that Black/African American children tend to be CMF victims more than other racial/ethnic groups; theory suggests that this is likely the result of racism—first, by increasing risk to children whose families experience racism at the societal and individual levels and second, through covert discrimination where professionals are more likely to identify a child of African descent as being victims of CMFs.
- Decades of research tells us that children die at the hands of their caregivers and most often, their mothers. Overall, women are more responsible for deaths that result from neglect and men are more responsible for deaths that result from abuse, but certainly both men and women can, and do, perpetrate all kinds of fatal maltreatment against children. This is well understood by researchers, but there is evidence that it is less well-known by child welfare professionals and perhaps the public at large.
- Children who die from maltreatment are more likely to live in households where non-family members are present.
- About one-third to one-half of children who die from maltreatment are known to child protective services.

3.4.2 What Remains Unknown

The field is less clear about everything else, which is a wide range of child and family characteristics; this includes child behavior, parent knowledge of child development, parent-child relationship, parental mental health or substance use, socioeconomic status, social isolation, domestic violence, and why victims are not reported to child protective services prior to death. There is research on bits and pieces of these characteristics, but as a whole, we lack definitive information which could guide social service providers to identify risk factors among children in the community, for child welfare professionals to conduct more effective risk assessments and for children to receive more impactful interventions. In truth, one of the reasons that this area of study is so difficult to examine is that all of the risk factors that I have addressed in this chapter for fatal maltreatment are also risk factors for non-fatal maltreatment.

At what point does a risk factor not only place a child at risk for abuse or neglect—which is bad enough in and of itself, but also place a child at risk for fatal maltreatment? This is question that cannot be answered at this time. Let's consider the case of being a "difficult child." The literature is fairly certain that children who are "difficult" are more likely to suffer a fatality at the hands of their caregivers. That said, being a difficult child is a risk factor for non-abusive harsh parenting and non-fatal maltreatment, in addition to fatal maltreatment. So far, it is unclear at what point being a difficult child puts one at-risk for receiving fatal parenting techniques, as opposed to less-than optimum parenting. One possibility is that it may not be a single factor alone which places a child at-risk, but rather a constellation of risk factors and characteristics—like the study that found that child behavior problems, in combination with parental stress place a child at-risk for fatality (Graham et al., 2010). Similarly, another scholar (McKee, 2006) proposes a "risk matrix" in which he considers risk and protective factors for filicide, examining how a constellation of risk factors in combination with insufficient protective factors, can tip the scale toward a fatal outcome. In perhaps the most important study on risk factors for CMF to date, one set of researchers examined what constellation of perpetrator risk factors ends in an abusive fatality (Yampolskaya et al., 2009). Using a sample of fatal and non-fatal maltreatment, the authors identified three classes of perpetrators, (1) birth mothers with physical and mental health problems, (2) male perpetrators with a history of domestic violence perpetration, who are less likely to be the birth parent and who are somewhat older, and (3) multiple problem perpetrators, where almost two-thirds were male, birth parents, living with the victims, and had problems in the area of substance abuse, criminal background, and domestic violence perpetration. Using these groupings, the male perpetrators with a history of domestic violence were most likely to fatally assault the victims, followed by multiple-problem perpetrators, and last mothers with health problems. Qualitative researchers, in their detailed examination of women who are incarcerated for the deaths of their children, have also painted pictures of families that are marked with chaos, mobility, poverty, abuse, and low knowledge of child development (Korbin, 1987, 1989, 1998; Oberman & Meyer, 2008). These studies have primarily focused on children who died from abuse, as opposed to neglect, but they serve as a model for where future research needs to take us, which is to understand when a constellation of child and family characteristics create an environment toxic enough for children that it costs them their lives.

References

Anderson, R., Ambrosino, R., Valentine, D., & Lauderdale, M. (1983). Child deaths attributed to abuse and neglect: An empirical study. *Children and Youth Services Review, 5*(1), 75–89.

Anyon, Y. (2011). Reducing racial disparities and disproportionalities in the child welfare system: Policy perspectives about how to serve the best interests of African American youth. *Children and Youth Services Review, 33*(2), 242–253. doi:10.1016/j.childyouth.2010.09.007.

Berlin, L. J., Appleyard, K., & Dodge, K. A. (2011). Intergenerational continuity in child maltreatment: Mediating mechanisms and implications for prevention. *Child Development, 82*(1), 162–176.

Beveridge, J. (1994). Analysis of Colorado child maltreatment fatalities. *Colorado's Children, 13*(2), 3–6.

Blackson, T. C., Tarter, R. E., & Maezzich, A. C. (1996). Interaction between childhood temperament and parental discipline practices on behavioral adjustment in preadolescent sons of substance abuse and normal fathers. *American Journal of Drug and Alcohol Abuse, 22*(3), 335–348.

Brewster, A. L., Nelson, J. P., Hymel, K. P., Colby, D. R., Lucas, D. R., McCanne, T. R., & Milner, J. S. (1998). Victim, perpetrator, family, and incident characteristics of 32 infant maltreatment deaths in the United States Air Force. *Child Abuse & Neglect, 22*(2), 91–101. doi:http://dx.doi.org/10.1016/S0145-2134(97)00132-4.

Carrier, P. (2002, June 27). Lawmakers vow vigilance on DHS; In the wake of the Schofield trial, they want to make sure child-welfare reforms are fully implemented. *Portland Press Herald*, p. 1A.

Casady, M. (2013, October 13). A "suspicious" death probed. *San Antonio Express News*. Retrieved from http://www.expressnews.com/news/local/article/A-suspicious-death-probed-4891499.php

Cavanagh, K., Dobash, R. E., & Dobash, R. P. (2007). The murder of children by fathers in the context of child abuse. *Child Abuse & Neglect, 31*(7), 731–746. doi:10.1016/j.chiabu.2006.12.016.

Chance, T. C., & Scannapieco, M. (2002). Ecological correlates of child maltreatment: Similarities and differences between child fatality and nonfatality cases. *Child and Adolescent Social Work Journal, 19*(2), 139–161.

Child Maltreatment Research Listserv. (2009, August 25). [New bulletin: Updated Trends in Child Maltreatment, 2008].

Clark, P., Buchanan, J., & Legters, L. (2008). Taking action on racial disproportionality in the child welfare system. *Child Welfare: Journal of Policy, Practice, and Program, 87*(2), 319–334.

Crofoot, T. L., & Harris, M. S. (2012). An Indian Child Welfare perspective on disproportionality in child welfare. *Children and Youth Services Review, 34*(9), 1667–1674. doi:10.1016/j.childyouth.2012.04.028.

Cross, T. L. (2008). Disproportionality in child welfare. *Child Welfare: Journal of Policy, Practice, and Program, 87*(2), 11–20.

Damashek, A., Nelson, M. M., & Bonner, B. L. (2013). Fatal child maltreatment: Characteristics of deaths from physical abuse versus neglect. *Child Abuse & Neglect, 37*(10), 735–744. doi:http://dx.doi.org/10.1016/j.chiabu.2013.04.014.

Davis, D. (Writer). (1987). The unquiet death of Eli Creekmore. In K. T. Seattle (Producer). USA.

Delsordo, J. D., & Leavitt, J. (1974). *Protective casework for abused children.* Morristown, NJ: General Learning Corporation.

Dettlaff, A. J., & Rycraft, J. R. (2008). Deconstructing disproportionality: Views from multiple community stakeholders. *Child Welfare: Journal of Policy, Practice, and Program, 87*(2), 37–58.

Douglas, E. M. (2012). Child welfare workers' training, knowledge, and practice concerns regarding child maltreatment fatalities: An exploratory, multi-state analysis. *Journal of Public Child Welfare, 6*(5), 659–677. doi:10.1080/15548732.2012.723975.

Douglas, E. M. (2013). Case, service and family characteristics of households that experience a child maltreatment fatality in the United States. *Child Abuse Review, 22*(5), 311–326. doi:10.1002/car.2236.

Douglas, E. M. (2016). Testing if social services prevent fatal child maltreatment among a sample of children previously known to child protective services. *Child Maltreatment.* doi:10.1177/1077559516657890.

Douglas, E. M., & Mohn, B. L. (2014). Fatal and non-fatal child maltreatment in the US: An analysis of child, caregiver, and service utilization with the National Child Abuse and Neglect Data Set. *Child Abuse & Neglect, 38*(1), 42–51. doi:http://dx.doi.org/10.1016/j.chiabu.2013.10.022.

Drake, B., Jolley, J. M., Lanier, P., Fluke, J., Barth, R. P., & Jonson-Reid, M. (2011). Racial bias in child protection? A comparison of competing explanations using national data. *Pediatrics, 127*(3), 471–478. doi:10.1542/peds.2010-1710.

Dretzin, R., Goodman, B., & Soenens, M. (Writers). (2003). Part I, The Taking of Logan Marr. In Frontline (Producer), Failure to protect: Public Broadcasting System.

Engfer, A., & Schneewind, K. (1982). Causes and consequences of harsh parental punishment: An empirical investigation in a representative sample of 570 German families. *Child Abuse and Neglect, 6*(2), 129–139.

Fein, L. G. (1979). Can child fatalities, end product child abuse, be prevented? *Children and Youth Services Review, 1,* 31–53.

Foster, C. H. (2012). Race and child welfare policy: State-level variations in disproportionality. *Race and Social Problems, 4*(2), 93–101. doi:10.1007/s12552-012-9071-9.

Gelles, R. J. (1973). Child abuse as psychopathology – A sociological critique and reformulation. *American Journal of Orthopsychiatry, 43*(4), 611–621.

Gelles, R. J. (1978). Profile of violence towards children in the United States. *American Journal of Orthopsychiatry, 48*(4), 580–592.

Gelles, R. J. (1996). *The book of David: How preserving families can cost children's lives.* New York, NY: Basic Books.

Gelles, R. J., & Harrop, J. W. (1991). The risk of abusive violence among children with nongenetic caretakers. *Family Relations, 40*(1), 78–83.

George, C., & Main, M. (1979). Social interactions of young abused children: Approach, avoidance, and aggression. *Child Development, 50*(2), 306–318. doi:10.2307/1129405.

Graham, J. C., Stepura, K., Baumann, D. J., & Kern, H. (2010). Predicting child fatalities among less-severe CPS investigations. *Children and Youth Services Review, 32*(2), 274–280. doi:10.1016/j.childyouth.2009.09.006.

Hamilton, L. R. (1989). Variables associated with child maltreatment and implications for prevention and treatment. *Early Child Development and Care, 42,* 31–56. doi:10.1080/0300443890420103.

Herman-Giddens, M. E., Smith, J. B., Mittal, M., Carlson, M., & Butts, J. D. (2003). Newborns killed or left to die by a parent: A population-based study. *JAMA, 289*(11), 1425–1429.

Jason, J., & Andereck, N. D. (1983). Fatal child abuse in Georgia: The epidemiology of severe physical child abuse. *Child Abuse & Neglect, 7*(1), 1–9. doi:10.1016/0145-2134(83)90023-6.

Jonson-Reid, M., Chance, T., & Drake, B. (2007). Risk of death among children reported for non-fatal maltreatment. *Child Maltreatment, 12*(1), 86–95. doi:10.1177/1077559506296722.

Kajese, T. M., Nguyen, L. T., Pham, G. Q., Pham, V. K., Melhorn, K., & Kallail, K. J. (2011). Characteristics of child abuse homicides in the state of Kansas from 1994 to 2007. *Child Abuse & Neglect, 35*(2), 147–154. doi:10.1016/j.chiabu.2010.11.002.

Klevens, J., & Leeb, R. T. (2010). Child maltreatment fatalities in children under 5: Findings from the National Violence Death Reporting System. *Child Abuse & Neglect, 34*(4), 262–266.

Knott, T., & Donovan, K. (2010). Disproportionate representation of African-American children in foster care: Secondary analysis of the national child abuse and neglect data system, 2005. *Children and Youth Services Review, 32*(5), 679–684.

Knott, T., & Giwa, S. (2012). African American disproportionality within CPS and disparate access to support services: Review and critical analysis of the literature. *Residential Treatment for Children & Youth, 29*(3), 219–230. doi:10.1080/0886571x.2012.697434.

Korbin, J. E. (1987). Incarcerated mothers' perceptions and interpretations of their fatally maltreated children. *Child Abuse & Neglect, 11*, 397–407.

Korbin, J. E. (1989). Fatal maltreatment by mothers: A proposed framework. *Child Abuse & Neglect, 13*(4), 481–489. doi:http://dx.doi.org/10.1016/0145-2134(89)90052-5.

Korbin, J. E. (1998). "Good mothers," "Babykillers" and fatal child maltreatment. In N. Scheper-Hughes & C. Sargent (Eds.), *Small wars: The cultural politics of childhood* (pp. 253–276). Berkeley, CA/Los Angeles, CA: University of California Press.

Kunz, J., & Bahr, S. J. (1996). A profile of parental homicide against children. *Journal of Family Violence, 11*(4), 347–362.

Levine, M., Freeman, J., & Compaan, C. (1994). Maltreatment-related fatalities: Issues of policy and prevention. *Law & Policy, 16*(4), 449–471.

Levitzky, S., & Cooper, R. (2000). Infant colic syndrome – Maternal fantasies of aggression and infanticide. *Clinical Pediatrics, 39*(7), 395–400. doi:10.1177/000992280003900703.

Lucas, D. R., Wezner, K. C., Milner, J. S., McCanne, T. H. R., Harris, I. N., Monroe-Posey, C., et al. (2002). Victim, perpetrator, family, and incident characteristics of infant and child homicide in the United States Air Force. *Child Abuse & Neglect, 26*, 167–186.

Manlove, E. E., & Vernon-Feagans, L. (2002). Caring for infant daughters and sons in dual-earner households: Maternal reports of father involvement in weekday time and tasks. *Infant & Child Development, 11*(4), 305–320.

Mapp, S. C. (2006). The effects of sexual abuse as a child on the risk of mothers physically abusing their children: A path analysis using systems theory. *Child Abuse & Neglect, 30*(11), 1293–1310.

Margolin, L. (1990). Fatal child neglect. *Child Welfare, 69*(4), 309–319.

Martin, J. A., Hamilton, B. E., Ventura, S. J., Osterman, M. J. K., Wilson, E. C., & Matthews, T. J. (2012). *Births: Final data for 2010 National Vital Statistical Reports* (Vol. 61).

McKee, G. R. (2006). *Why mothers kill: A forensic psychologist's casebook*. New York, NY: Oxford University Press.

Meyer, C., Oberman, M., & Rone, M. (2001). *Mothers who kill their children: Understanding the acts of moms from Susan Smith to the "prom mom"*. New York, NY: New York University Press.

Miller, C. M., & Burch, A. D. S. (2013a, August 18). Girl 2, pays with her life for DCF's inaction. *Miami Herald*. Retrieved from http://www.dailymail.co.uk/news/article-2397606/Florida-mother-Chelsea-Huggett-killed-disabled-daughter-Aliyah-Marie-Branum-2.html

Miller, C. M., & Burch, A. D. S. (2013b, August 20). Names of dead children invoked at hearing to reform DCF. *Miami Herald*. Retrieved from http://www.miamiherald.com/2013/08/20/3575635/names-of-dead-children-invoked.html-storylink=cpy

O'Malley, S. (2004). *Are you there alone? The unspeakable crime of Andrea Yates*. New York, NY: Simon & Schuster.

Oberman, M., & Meyer, C. L. (2008). *When mothers kill: Interviews from prison*. New York, NY: New York University Press.

Palusci, V. J., & Covington, T. M. (2014). Child maltreatment deaths in the U.S. National Child Death Review Case Reporting System. *Child Abuse & Neglect, 38*(1), 25–36. doi:http://dx.doi.org/10.1016/j.chiabu.2013.08.014.

Paulozzi, L. (2002). Variation in homicide risk during infancy – United States, 1989–1998. *Morbidity and Mortality Weekly Report, 51*(9), 189–189.

Sabotta, E. E., & Davis, R. L. (1992). Fatality after report to a child abuse registry in Washington state, 1973–1986. *Child Abuse & Neglect, 16*(5), 627–635.

Schnitzer, P. G., & Ewigman, B. G. (2008). Household composition and fatal unintentional injuries related to child maltreatment. *Journal of Nursing Scholarship, 40*(1), 91–97.

Sherrod, K. B., Altemeier, W. A., O'Connor, S., & Vietze, P. M. (1984). Early prediction of child maltreatment. *Early Child Development and Care, 13*(3–4), 335–350.

Sinal, S. H., Petree, A. R., Herman-Giddens, M., Rogers, M. K., Enand, C., & DuRant, R. H. (2000). Is race or ethnicity a predictive factor in shaken baby syndrome? *Child Abuse & Neglect, 24*(9), 1241–1246. doi:10.1016/s0145-2134(00)00177-0.

Sinha, V., Trocmé, N., Fallon, B., & MacLaurin, B. (2013). Understanding the investigation-stage overrepresentation of first nations children in the child welfare system: An analysis of the first nations component of the Canadian incidence study of reported child abuse and neglect 2008. *Child Abuse & Neglect.* doi:10.1016/j.chiabu.2012.11.010.

Stiffman, M. N., Schnitzer, P. G., Adam, P., Kruse, R. L., & Ewigman, B. G. (2002). Household composition and risk of fatal child maltreatment. *Pediatrics, 109*(4), 615–621. doi:10.1542/peds.109.4.615.

Stith, S. M., Liu, T., Davies, L. C., Boykin, E. L., Alder, M. C., Harris, J. M., … Dees, J. E. M. E. G. (2009). Risk factors in child maltreatment: A meta-analytic review of the literature. *Aggression and Violent Behavior, 14*(1), 13–29.

Tourigny, J. A. (2006). *High-risk environments and infant health: Predicting psychological and physical health outcomes with maternal, child, and parenting variables.* Doctorate, University of Saskatchewan, Canada.

U.S. Department of Health & Human Services. (2011). *Child maltreatment 2010: Reports from the States to the National Child Abuse and Neglect Data Systems – National statistics on child abuse and neglect.* Washington, DC: Administration for Children & Families, U.S. Department of Health & Human Services.

U.S. Department of Health & Human Services. (2012). *Child maltreatment 2011: Reports from the States to the National Child Abuse and Neglect Data Systems – National statistics on child abuse and neglect.* Washington, DC: Administration for Children & Families, U.S. Department of Health & Human Services.

U.S. Department of Health & Human Services. (2013). *Child maltreatment 2012: Reports from the States to the National Child Abuse and Neglect Data Systems – National statistics on child abuse and neglect.* Washington, DC: Administration for Children & Families, U.S. Department of Health & Human Services.

U.S. Department of Health & Human Services. (2014). *Child maltreatment 2013: Reports from the States to the National Child Abuse and Neglect Data Systems – National statistics on child abuse and neglect.* Washington, DC: Administration for Children & Families, U.S. Department of Health & Human Services.

U.S. Department of Health & Human Services. (2015). *Child maltreatment 2014: Reports from the States to the National Child Abuse and Neglect Data Systems – National statistics on child abuse and neglect.* Washington, DC: Administration for Children & Families, U.S. Department of Health & Human Services.

Welch, G. L., & Bonner, B. L. (2013). Fatal child neglect: Characteristics, causation, and strategies for prevention. *Child Abuse & Neglect, 37*(10), 745–752. doi:http://dx.doi.org/10.1016/j.chiabu.2013.05.008.

Whipple, E. E. (1999). Reaching families with preschoolers at risk of physical child abuse: What works? *Families in Society, 80*(2), 148–160.

Wood, J. J., & Repetti, R. L. (2004). What gets dad involved? A longitudinal study of change in parental child caregiving involvement. *Journal of Family Psychology, 18*(1), 237–249.

World Health Organization. (2001). *Comparative risk assessment: Child sexual abuse.* Sydney, Australia: WHO Collaborating Centre for Evidence and Health Policy in Mental Health.

Yampolskaya, S., Greenbaum, P. E., & Berson, I. R. (2009). Profiles of child maltreatment perpetrators and risk for fatal assault: A latent class analysis. *Journal of Family Violence, 24*(5), 337–348.

Chapter 4
The Intersection of the Child Welfare Profession and Maltreatment Fatalities

Most of the research on child maltreatment fatalities (CMFs) and the child welfare profession has focused on the aftermath—how having a child killed or die on one's caseload changes workers, supervisors, and managers, and the emotional toll that it takes on workers who are directly or indirectly affected by the death (Ayre, 2001; Douglas, 2009; Gustavsson & MacEachron, 2004; Horwath, 1995; Regehr, Chau, Leslie, & Howe, 2002). Instances where a child dies when s/he was previously known to child protective services have also been linked to the development of a culture of blame and mistrust in child protection work (Lachman & Bernard, 2006) and to an increase in policing functions of child welfare professionals (Regehr et al., 2002). Further, the professional literature is rich with discussions about how to support workers after a critical incident and how the death of a child provides an opportunity for learning and change (Csikai, Herrin, Tang, & Church Ii, 2008; Gustavsson & MacEachron, 2004). The field, however, has been relatively silent on how to prevent CMFs within the child welfare profession and which workers might be more likely to experience a fatality. There has been substantial discussion about improved risk assessment tools and how to make decisions made by child welfare workers (CWWs) more objective and less subjective (Arad-Davidzon & Benbenishty, 2008; Baumann, Law, Sheets, Reid, & Graham, 2005; Regehr, Bogo, Shlonsky, & LeBlanc, 2010; Shlonsky & Wagner, 2005), but rarely has this discussion been linked to fatalities in a tangible way.

This book focuses on the policy, programmatic, and other professional responses to fatal child maltreatment and whether the actions that we have taken have improved circumstances and outcomes for children. The creation of the child welfare profession couldn't be described as a policy or programmatic response to fatal child maltreatment alone, but it is shaped by the crisis that follows fatalities. Further, there is no other professional group that is in the unique position of preventing fatalities from abuse and neglect. The child welfare profession largely engages in the tertiary prevention of child maltreatment, meaning that workers respond to instances of abuse and neglect that have already occurred or where imminent risk of harm is present (see Chapter 1). This means that CWWs should be uniquely positioned to prevent the worst outcomes of maltreatment—the death of a child. In other words, child welfare professionals are in the child fatality prevention business—something that is not usually discussed or described in the professional literature or on the ground in the field. My work in this area shows that workers are inadequately prepared to prevent children from dying from maltreatment. Thus, in this chapter, the book takes a turn and begins to focus on the policies, programs, and professional responses that are in place today to prevent CMFs. I start with the most obvious place—the child welfare profession itself. In this particular chapter I focus on workers' concerns, training, and knowledge around CMFs, and then discuss workers who experienced the death of a child and briefly touch on how workers respond to the deaths of these clients. Finally, I speculate on how workers might miss warning signs leading up to the fatality. As with other chapters in this book, I highlight the controversies throughout this chapter, but also note them here as well.

- Workers have significant gaps in knowledge about risk factors for CMFs
- Workers who have a child die on their caseload appear to be experienced workers with adequate education and work experience
- There is a potential disconnect between using a strengths perspective in child welfare practice while also assessing for risk factors for maltreatment.

4.1 Child Maltreatment Fatalities: Perceptions and Experiences of Child Welfare Professionals Study

From September 2010 to January 2011, I conducted a study about the intersection of CWWs and fatal maltreatment. Because it is the only large-scale study on this topic, my findings will be the basis for most of this chapter. In this online study, I recruited 426 child welfare professionals from 25 states to participate; 123 (27.2%) had experienced a maltreatment fatality on their caseload. I recruited participants through advertisement on professional websites, social media sites targeting social workers, child maltreatment listservs, and through direct appeals to child welfare agency administrators. The purpose of the study was to assess the knowledge, attitudes, practice concerns, and experiences with maltreatment fatalities among U.S. child welfare professionals. The findings of this study have been published in a number of separate papers, which are cited throughout the chapter.

4.1.1 CWWs' Knowledge, Practice Concerns, and Opinions About CMFs

4.1.1.1 Practice Concerns and Opinions

In general, CWWs are concerned that a child on their caseload will die from maltreatment (Douglas, 2012). Almost three-quarters (72%) of workers in this sample worried that a child on their caseload will die and the vast majority (93%) reported assessing for risk of fatality when they work with families. One worker's description of the profession's work, worry, and concern captures this sentiment especially well:

> "The blame for a child death usually lands on the frontline worker. We can not [sic] live with the families we work with. While a good service worker can prevent some maltreatment, it is impossible to prevent all maltreatment. In some situations workers do not have the evidence needed to legally mandate a family into services which might prevent maltreatment. As a worker I am extremely stressed out by my caseload and frequently worry that a child will die. I work weekends and sometimes until 8 or 9 pm to keep up with the work but if one child dies I will never feel that I did enough. Most CWWs truly care about the families on their caseloads but preventing maltreatment while keeping up with 20 to 30 investigations is impossible. We are fighting a losing battle…My entire academic experience as a professional social worker has prepared me for this job and I am still overwhelmed by the massive responsibility."

A substantial proportion of workers, 28%, had a parent disclose a potential intent to kill his/her child. This is the first time that this practice event has been measured, thus it is impossible to know if this finding is consistent with other research. The finding is, however, concerning and speaks to many of the high-risk and complex family situations that child welfare professionals encounter.

The survey also asked workers for some of their opinions about CMFs. For example, I asked workers if they thought that children who died were "the same" as children who did not die, and that CMF is a freak event that could happen to any child involved in the child welfare system. Almost 40% of workers agreed with this statement. This question was included as an opinion because there is limited research about the extent to which children who die are "the same" or "different." That said, there is some research, which in comparing fatal and non-fatal victims and families who are involved with the child welfare system has found that children who are killed are seen as being more difficult than children who do not die (Chance & Scannapieco, 2002; Graham, Stepura, Baumann, & Kern, 2010) (see Chapter 3 for more information). This might be an indicator that children who die are indeed "different," at least, according to their parents. This particular finding may have important implications for child welfare practice.

One significant concern that emerges from this finding is that workers who believe that a CMF is a freak occurrence may be less likely to see themselves as agents of prevention, less likely to assess for risk, and to take action when it is warranted. Further, the professional literature supports a positive relationship between attitudes/beliefs of CWWs and their practice behaviors in the field (Arad-Davidzon & Benbenishty, 2008; Smith, 2008); for example, workers who feel more positively about removal a child from a birth parent is more likely to do so. This area of child welfare practice is in need of additional research; I recommend focusing on the attitudes of CWWs and how those attitudes potentially translate into how a worker formulates or conceptualizes a case, and how it relates to actions taken to protect children.

4.1.2 CWWs' Knowledge of Risk Factors for CMFs

One of the key areas of this study was to examine workers' level of knowledge about risk factors for maltreatment fatalities. I presented a series of statements about risk factors for CMFs, some of which were accurate and some of which were not. I asked workers to indicate the extent to which they agreed with each statement, as it relates to CMFs. I found that there is a wide range of knowledge in this area. Workers were most knowledgeable about children's age as a risk factor and also that parents of fatality victims often have age-inappropriate expectations of their children. Workers had considerably less knowledge concerning parental and perpetrator risk factors. Only 20% of workers knew that mothers are most responsible for their children's deaths; only 38% knew that children are most likely to be killed by a family member (as compared with a non-family member); and only 42% knew that more children die from neglect. Figure 4.1[1] shows the full results of workers' level of knowledge.

The results of these analyses indicate that workers appear to think that children are most commonly killed by non-family members; further, less than half knew that more children die from neglect. Research on risk factors for CMFs is still developing, but as I discussed in Chapter 3, two of the most consistent findings of research on child welfare-related fatalities are that mothers are most often the perpetrators of maltreatment fatalities and that the most common cause of death is neglect.[2] CWWs had more knowledge about the risks of the parent-child relationship, such as whether parents describe their children as being difficult. At least 71% of the sample accurately identified parent-child characteristics that would be considered risks. Workers had less knowledge of household risk factors, however. Between one-third to one-half of the sample was inaccurate at some point in their assessment of household risk factors, such as having non-family members living in a house or family mobility.

An easy conclusion would be to decide that the child welfare system is failing. A fairer assessment would be to ask to what extent professionals in other fields are knowledgeable about risk factors for other types of child fatalities. The findings are not encouraging. For example, only 20% of night-time childcare centers follow the recommendations of the Centers for Disease Control and Prevention about placing babies on their backs, as opposed to their stomachs to sleep; the so-called "back-to-sleep" campaign (Moon, Weese-Mayer, & Silvestri, 2003). Similarly, a study of health providers found that almost two-thirds of the sample reported not knowing the causes of or strategies for preventing still births (Ojofeitimi et al., 2009). Research suggests that physicians' have a limited understanding of the suicidal risks

---

[1] The wording in Figure 4.1 is not the exact wording that was used in the questionnaire. The wording has been summarized for ease of display in a table.

[2] In the survey I used the word "kill:" "Mothers are the ones who are most likely to kill their children." It is possible that workers interpreted the word "kill" to mean action, as opposed to inaction. If the question had been phrased "Mothers are most often responsible for the deaths of their children," it is possible that respondents may have answered differently.

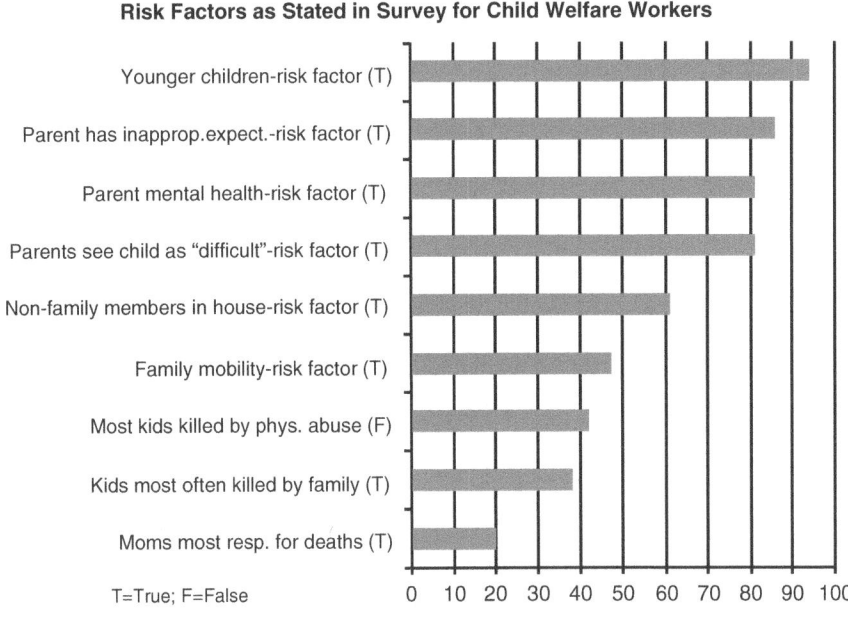

Figure 4.1 Worker Knowledge of Risk Factors for Maltreatment Fatalities. Adapted from Douglas, E. M. (2012). CWWs' training, knowledge, and practice concerns regarding child maltreatment fatalities: An exploratory, multi-state analysis. *Journal of Public Child Welfare, 6*(5), 659–677

associated with youth taking antidepressants (Cordero, Rudd, Bryan, & Corso, 2008); further, community providers' often have limited knowledge about the facts and risk factors for youth suicide (Baber & Bean, 2009). Thus, CWWs are not alone in their limited knowledge about risk factors for fatalities. That said, the limits of other fields do not justify the ill preparedness of CWWs. In short, the findings provide compelling evidence for workers to receive more training around risk factors for maltreatment deaths.

4.1.3 Training About CMFs

The fact that workers were more likely to think that most children die from abuse, as opposed to neglect, and are killed by non-family, as opposed to family members, suggests that workers are "getting their training" about CMFs along with the rest of the public—in the media. Cases of CMF that make it into the media are usually those that are most prosecutable—involving physical abuse and often a non-parent caregiver. One would imagine that workers receive training about risk factors for CMFs, but in truth, the question had never been asked or pursued within the professional literature before. So, the results of this study on CWWs prompted two other studies that I conducted with colleagues concerning the preparation for being a child welfare worker.

In one study we examined 24 child welfare, child abuse and neglect, and other child-based text books and looked for content around CMFs (Douglas & Serino, 2013). Specifically, we wanted to know if textbooks which future CWWs might read contained information about CMFs, if they listed risk factors for CMFs, and if so, if the information presented was accurate. We found that the majority of textbooks (70–75%, n = 17 or 18) contained information on CMFs: a definition, the ways that children die, and who is responsible for children's deaths. There was, however, considerably less information about incidence rates, as well as child, parent, and household/family risk factors in the books that we reviewed. For example, of the 24 books, only seven stated that more children die from neglect than abuse. The most frequently cited risk factor for children was age, but even then, only 14 of the 24 books provided this information. Even less frequently cited, this time by ten books, was the fact that being described as a "difficult child" increases the risk for CMF victimization. Other child risk factors were only mentioned by a handful of books. Some mentioned factors that place a child at risk for non-fatal maltreatment, but for which there is insufficient evidence concerning fatal maltreatment. The inclusion of parental risk factors was even lower than child risk factors. Parental mental health concerns were mentioned in ten textbooks. The remaining parental risk factors, including that mothers are most often responsible for CMFs, was mentioned in only five to eight books. With regard to family/household risk factors, family unemployment was cited most often, by eight books. Our review and analysis of CMF content in social science textbooks shows that authors of books on child abuse and neglect or child welfare, do not include substantive information about CMFs or the risk factors that increase the likelihood that children will die and sometimes include information that is false, stands as speculation, or is not fully confirmed by research.

In the next study, two colleagues and I examined the pre-service training curricula that are offered to CWWs before they begin working in the field (Douglas, Mohn, & Gushwa, 2015). The content and length of each curriculum is decided by individual states and child welfare agencies or partnering agencies. We collected the pre-service training curricula from 20 states and, like the previous study on textbooks, examined them for content about CMFs—definitions, descriptions of causes of death, perpetrators, prevalence rates, and risk factors. Of the 20 curricula reviewed, ten made reference to child maltreatment fatalities: one provided a case example; one provided a definition for child maltreatment fatality; three documented statistics related to CMFs; seven mentioned risk factors associated with CMFs, and four curricula cited CMFs as being caused by neglect more than abuse. Florida is the only state that included a full section on CMFs. There was little information provided to new CWWs about CMFs. The information that was most widely available centered on the fact that young children are at an increased risk for fatality, which was presented by four states. We did not find evidence of inaccurate information, as we did in the review of textbooks.

In my research on CWWs and maltreatment fatalities, I did inquire about whether workers had received training about maltreatment fatalities. Despite what my colleagues and I learned about pre-service training curricula, almost three-quarters (73%) of the sample reported having received training on CMFs. It is not clear if this training was provided during pre-service training or through special workshops or conferences at other points in their careers; the duration and depth of the training is also unknown. As noted before, the professional literature has addressed child welfare training in general (Antle, Frey, Sar, Barbee, & van Zyl, 2009; Franke, Bagdasaryan, & Furman, 2009; Keys, 2009), but nothing that is about CMFs or high-risk families.

The unfortunate news is that the training did not appear to make any difference in workers' knowledge about or of risk factors for CMFs. The only real difference between workers who had been trained and those who had not—with regard to knowledge of risk factors—concerned workers' knowledge of parental mental health problems as a risk factor for fatality. Workers who had received training were *less likely* to accurately identify this as a risk—not an outcome that one would hope to find. Even more concerning, only 14% of the workers in this study reported feeling insecure in their level of knowledge concerning risk factors for fatality, despite gaps in their understanding of risk factors. Further, workers who had received training were more likely to have confidence in their knowledge, yet the results showed overall, high levels of inaccurate "knowledge."

There are a few glimmers of hope in this sea of bad news about training and knowledge of risk factors. One, the vast majority of workers (90%) reported wanting more training about risk factors for fatalities. Two, the child welfare profession, in general, is increasing research on the effectiveness of training (Collins, Amodeo, & Clay, 2008; Curry, McCarragher, & Dellmann-Jenkins, 2005; Franke et al., 2009); this is an area that deserves increased attention from scholars and practitioners.

4.2 Workers Who Experience the Death of a Child Client

Research has shown that between 30 and 50% (Anderson, Ambrosino, Valentine, & Lauderdale, 1983; Beveridge, 1994; Damashek, Nelson, & Bonner 2013) of children who die from a maltreatment fatality were previously known or their families were previously known to their state/county's child welfare agency before their death. Statistics from 2012 indicate that in 8.5% of cases of CMFs, families had received family preservation services in the 5 years before the death, and 2.2% of CMF cases, families had received reunification services in the 5 years before the death. In addition to these services, children and their families could have received support services or been the subject of a report that was screened out.

Annually, a fair number of workers have experience with fatalities. For example, if 30–50% of children who die each year are known to child welfare agencies that means that in 2012, when 1,592 children died from maltreatment, between 477 and 796 of these victims or their families had contact with child welfare services before they died. Since every child has a worker and a supervisor, this means that between 954 and 1,592 child welfare professionals experienced a fatality on their caseload in 2012. Using the *Child Maltreatment* report of the 2012 data (see Chapter 2), I estimate that there are 35,716 CWWs in the United States (U.S. Department of Health & Human Services, 2013). Thus, I further estimate that between 2.7 and 4.5% of the child welfare workforce has an experience with a child dying on his or her caseload. (This estimate may be slightly inflated because multiple children sometimes die in a single family, who would have had a single worker.) To put this into context, this means that more workers experience the death of a child client due to maltreatment than all of the workers in the one state of Arizona.

CMFs have often been attributed to inexperienced workers who are assigned to high risk cases; a report by the Los Angeles County (California) Children's Special Investigation Unit pointed to lack of experience as a contributing factor to the deaths of 15 children in 2010–2011 (County of Los Angeles Children's Special Investigation Unit, 2012). A special investigation's report described emergency child welfare work as: "[W]orkers who are skilled and experienced are the least likely to opt for an ER assignment…ER workers are more likely to be inexperienced, overworked, and just 'doing time' before moving on to a more desirable assignment" (pp. 18–19). Some members of academia have spoken negatively about the child welfare system and how it employs workers who are young, lack education and training, and how these factors might place children at higher risk for fatality (Gelles, 2003).

Similar conclusions have been drawn by the media (Batty, 2001) and organizations with a mission to reform the child welfare system (National Coalition for Child Protection Reform, 2009): "These untrained, inexperienced workers with overwhelming caseloads are sent out to make life and death decisions" (p. 1).

These popular and anecdotal descriptions of CWWs are not consistent with what I found in the sample of workers who volunteered to participate in my study. For those workers who had experienced a CMF on their caseload, I asked about their age, experience, and education at the time of the death. I also asked about the size of their caseload and their approach to the case prior to the fatality. I found that the CWWs who experienced a CMF on their caseload were in their 30s and well trained; specifically, I found that frontline workers were, on average 35 years old and supervisors were 41. This would place workers, age-wise, in middle adulthood and mid-career. Overall, the professionals had been in the field an average of 6 years, with frontline workers averaging 4 years at the time of the fatality and supervisors averaging 13 years. Collectively, 98% had a college degree and over half (52%) had a master's degree. Over half of the sample (60%) had a degree in social work or human services and another 29% had a degree in another social science. Only 11% had a degree in a discipline outside of the social sciences. These findings do not describe a group of CWWs who are young, uneducated, or underprepared for the rigors of child welfare casework. In fact, as compared to a nationally, representative sample of CWWs, they are on par with, or have more experience, more relevant education, and a higher level of education at the time that the fatality occurred (Barth, Lloyd, Christ, Chapman, & Dickinson, 2008).

Workers who experienced a CMF had a median of 25 cases on their caseload and had carried the case that ended in a fatality on their load for about 2 months. The numbers of cases that the workers were carrying are not grossly outside of what is recommended by the Child Welfare League of America—the nation's leading professional association for the child welfare profession. The League states that frontline workers should not handle more than 17 cases, and that supervisors should not handle more than 85 cases (Child Welfare League of America, 1999). In my study, frontline workers who had a child die had 20 cases and supervisors had 90. These additional cases might have been enough to compromise the workers' job performance, but without research in this area, one can only speculate.

4.2.1 Handling of Case Prior to Fatality

I also asked workers about their handling of the case before the child died. I wondered—did they worry about the family more than usual? Did they want to do something different, but their supervisor or a policy prevent them from doing so? The vast majority of workers indicated that the case was proceeding as all of their cases proceed. A strong majority of the sample (78–84%) felt confident in the handling of the case prior to the CMF: workers felt that they received appropriate guidance, felt confident, and had not especially worried about the child/family. Only a minority (10–12%) reported wanting to pursue another course of action before the child died. Supervisors, as opposed to frontline workers, felt especially confident in having received appropriate guidance on the case. There is little research that addresses how confident workers feel in their jobs (Regehr et al., 2010; Strand & Bosco-Ruggiero, 2010). What exists shows that beginning social workers report feeling at least moderately confident to engage in child welfare practice (Jones & Okamura, 2000).

Finally, over a quarter of the CWWs who had a child die on their caseload (27%) reported that the CMF that occurred on their caseload was unavoidable. I conducted a follow-up set of analyses to examine if this response varied by the manner in which the child died (e.g., physical abuse versus physical neglect) and it did not. These kinds of attitudes may not be restricted to the child who died. They may carry into practice techniques as a worker, as well—believing in the inability to change the outcomes for the families with whom they work. Conversely, it may say more about a general lack of confidence in the services that the system provides. It is also interesting to compare this result with workers' overall assessment and approach to the case. For example, workers who reported that they received adequate guidance on the case were more likely to indicate that the death was unavoidable.[3] These findings raise important questions about training, expectations on the part of workers, and the extent to which they see themselves as agents of prevention.

In general, we can conclude that CWWs were satisfied with their performance in handling the case before the child died, they did not want to pursue a different service plan for the family and they received adequate guidance. One conclusion from these findings is that the results are consistent with the public perception that CWWs are unable to recognize when a child is in danger of dying from maltreatment. The results previously discussed in this chapter about lack of knowledge of risk factors would contribute to this perception as well. Another perspective is that workers either believe or are reporting on the events leading up to the child's death in a manner that protects them from acknowledging faulty judgment or other forms of wrong-doing, such as not visiting the child as mandated by federal statute. No one wants to believe that he or she may have missed opportunities to take protection action to shelter a child from harm.

4.2.2 How Do Workers Miss Red Flags?[4]

After a child's death occurs, there are multiple opportunities to review the case, to examine the circumstances leading up to the death. These opportunities are presented by the media, by internal reviews in child welfare services, and by multidisciplinary child death review teams (see Chapter 5 for more information). Much of the time, the cases are riddled with risk factors, red flags everywhere. When examined retrospectively, those red flags are obvious—glaring opportunities for intervention to prevent the death of a child. Thus, the question is—if the red flags are obvious after the child's death, why were they not obvious before the child died? One possible reason has already been addressed—workers are not especially knowledgeable of which risk factors contribute to fatalities and thus, cases are inadequately conceptualized from the beginning. As I write this chapter, the state of Massachusetts, for example, is currently in the middle of a CMF crisis. Child welfare work in this state was described as follows: "The high-risk cases, which involve allegations of serious physical or sexual abuse, are referred to social workers who investigate the safety of the child, while the lower-risk cases, which involve neglect, are given to social workers charged with strengthening families" (Levenson, 2015). This child welfare practice approach is not consistent with research which consistently shows that more children die from neglect than physical abuse.

---

[3] Workers were asked to indicate the extent to which they agreed with the following statement: "The death was unavoidable."

[4] I have talked about this issue with many academic and child welfare colleagues, but two have been most influential in helping me critically examine this problem. Sandra S. Hodge and Dr. Melinda K. Gushwa, thank you for your insights.

Widespread misinformation and confusion abound when it comes to maltreatment fatalities. I found that CWWs who experienced the death of a child on their caseload, did not feel that they should have pursued a different course of action with the family prior to the child's death. When I testified in October 2014 before the U.S. National Commission to Eliminate Child Abuse and Neglect Fatalities, a commissioner stated to me during testimony, that they have repeatedly heard that there is no difference between children in the child welfare system who die and those who don't—even though research shows otherwise. The inability to detect this difference before death may be one of the most important issues that we seek to resolve in the attempt to prevent future CMFs. In truth, it is not entirely possible to know why CWWs miss red flags, because there is no research that has been conducted in this area yet. Thus, I can only speculate by drawing from what literature does exist concerning child welfare practice and by using anecdotes from the field. We can start with the current foundation of the social work profession: the strengths-based approach (Rapp, Saleebey, & Sullivan, 2005; Saleebey, 1992). The strengths perspective is a values-based approach toward working with social work clients. It is focused on acknowledging the strengths that an individual may possess, for example talents, values, competencies, hopes, and possibilities. It requires finding these strengths, even when they may have become lost or distorted in the face of trauma or oppression. The strengths perspective also recognizes the role that larger systems—institutions, policies, and programs—may play in oppressing individuals, groups, or communities and to prevent them from realizing their talents or goals (Saleebey, 1996). The strengths approach is an alternative to traditional modes of social work that focused on psychopathology, disease, and deficits that needed to be fixed by experts (Graybeal, 2001; Siegal, Rapp, Kelliher, & Fisher, 1995; Weick, 2009). According to Dennis Saleebey (2009), the father of the strengths-based approach, there are six core principles of the strengths perspective.

1. "Every individual, group, family, and community has strength.
2. Trauma and abuse, illness and struggle may be injurious, but they may also be sources of challenge and opportunity.
3. Assume that you do not know the upper limits of the capacity to grow and change and take individual, group, and community aspirations seriously.
4. We best serve clients by collaborating with them.
5. Every environment is full of resources.
6. Caring, caretaking, and context" (pp. 15–18).

Massachusetts is in the middle of a fatal child maltreatment crisis and its governor and commissioner have just declared that the safety of children will be placed over the goal of strengthening a child (Scharfenberg & Miller, 2015). That said, the social work profession and social work educators have largely embraced the strengths perspective (Graybeal, 2001; Probst, 2010). It has become widely adopted throughout the social service (Brun & Rapp, 2001; Huebner, Jones, Miller, Custer, & Critchfield, 2006; Sheely & Bratton, 2010; Werrbach, 1996) and child welfare professions (Kemp, Marcenko, Lyons, & Kruzich, 2014; Lietz, 2011; Lietz & Rounds, 2009; Mapp, 2002), yet there is limited evidence that it is an effective social work practice technique (Staudt, Howard, & Drake, 2001). Many have acknowledged the difficulty of integrating this approach into child welfare practice (Bundy-Fazioli, Briar-Lawson, & Hardiman, 2009; Kemp et al., 2014), but there has been limited discussion about how to balance assessing for risk while also focusing on strengths (Kemp et al., 2014; Shlonsky & Wagner, 2005) or, partnering with families while also having to police them. It is possible that CWWs who had a child die on their caseload reported feeling that the case was "on track," because they were focused on the family's strengths rather than potential risks to the child. Given the overwhelming attention to the strengths perspective and the movement away from focusing on a client's "deficits" (Graybeal, 2001), to propose that risk factors might trump a family's perceived strengths, is a controversial idea.

Add to this new orientation, that the child welfare profession has also made significant strides in moving away from solely relying on clinical hunches or judgments, through the implementation of actuarial-based risk assessment tools (Camasso & Jagannathan, 1995; D'Andrade, Austin, & Benton, 2008; English & Pecora, 1994). Risk assessment tools allow workers to quantitatively score individual items pertaining to a child's level of risk and then sum those items for a total score, which indicates the child's overall level of risk. Risk assessment tools are not flawless, however. They are completed by professionals, who are making their own determinations of risk.

Risk assessment tools allow workers to override the total score. In such instances, workers believe that the scoring either over- or underestimates the risk presented to the child. This is how clinical judgment and risk assessment tools are used together. If a worker has been encouraged to focus on family strengths, she might be prone to overriding the total score to indicate a lower level of risk than what is actually posed to the child. For example, if a family has a history of child maltreatment, that risk factor will never go away; it will continue to stand regardless of the progress that a parent makes. A worker might be inclined to think that this past history inflates a parent's "true" risk if the parent is presently doing well. Overriding a risk assessment tool may also feel "right" to a worker, especially given research which shows that workers' own attitudes and values influence their assessment of risk presented to a child (Davidson-Arad & Benbenishty, 2010) and that workers who feel that parents have been forthcoming with them feel more confident in their own determination of level of risk (Regehr et al., 2010).

Finally, there is some anecdotal evidence that CWWs may not fully understand what constitutes a "strength." A child welfare professional confided to me that she and her colleagues routinely see confusion in case files about what constitutes a strength, a phenomenon which she and her colleagues jokingly call "strengths-based confusion." She reported seeing references to the family's "nice" neighborhood, home, or curtains—none of which has the potential to act in a protective capacity toward a child. Others in the child welfare profession have corroborated such stories. During a recent guest talk at a school of social work, a student with 20 years' experience as a CWW relayed to me that there is tremendous pressure placed on workers to find strengths in a family, even if the workers feel one is not present. Colleagues and I recently heard about cases in which children were experiencing significant risk to their physical well-being (one of them ended in fatality), but because the workers determined that there were strengths present in the family, it gave them the false impression that it was acceptable to dismiss the risk factors that were also present. These workers seemed to be operating under the principle that risk factors can be canceled out by identifying the presence of a strength—any strength.

I want to be clear to the readers that this section of my book is speculation. We don't know about the connection between using a strengths perspective in child welfare work and CMFs. But, we do know that workers are experiencing significant pressure to focus on family strengths, without the evidence base to support this practice (Staudt et al., 2001). Further, even in an era when there is significant national media attention to CMFs, I maintain that there are inadequate conversations about how to balance assessing for risk and strengths. In my review of the literature, I also have yet to identify any writings or empirical evidence about what constitutes or defines a strength. The approach that comes closest is assessing for specific parenting capacities, such as knowledge of child develop or how the parent views the job of caretaking (ACTION for Child Protection, 2010; American Psychological Association, 2013; Budd, 2005). If we do not define this term for CWWs, they are left to define this term on their own, which is an extremely risky proposition. Last, we need to better understand how workers' own attitudes shape how they integrate focusing on strengths, assessing for risk, and how supervisors can mediate this process. The field's lack of knowledge in this area is glaring and until the child welfare profession sorts out this conflict in child welfare practice, I suspect that children will continue to die because of our inability to give workers evidence-based tools to work with families and to protect children.

4.3 The Aftermath of Child Maltreatment Fatalities

The death of a child who was previously known to child welfare agencies is a catalyst for action which can result in both formal and informal changes in policy and practice. A common and universally accepted result is the swinging of the "child welfare pendulum"—which radiates through legislatures, agencies, right down to frontline workers. If a child dies in his/her birth home, the pendulum swings toward removing current and future child clients and placing them in foster care—generally called the "child safety" approach. If a child died in his/her foster home, the pendulum swings toward keeping current and future child clients with their birth families—generally called the "family preservation" approach (Gelles, 1996).

At the legislative level, previous research has shown that media attention to deaths among children who were known to child welfare services often results in new state-level child welfare legislation (Gainsborough, 2009) that is intended to prevent future fatalities (Douglas, 2009). At the agency-level, children's deaths that occur in birth homes can lead to an increase in the use of foster care and deaths that occur in foster homes can lead to an increase in the use of family preservation

(Gelles, 1996; Murphy, 1997). Media attention can have an important impact on the climate of child welfare agencies. Cooper (2005) found that in an effort to improve accountability, management responded to media coverage by restricting the independence of frontline workers. Others also found that agency-related CMFs resulted in restricted practices and an increase in policing functions within a child welfare agency (Regehr et al., 2002). A British study noted that high profile CMFs resulted in a significant change in oversight procedures which had a deleterious effect on the overall atmosphere of the agency (Ayre, 2001).

After the death of a child client many agencies conduct internal reviews to identify what went wrong, who might be responsible, and how they can learn from any mistakes that were made. Workers often feel distressed by the repeated exposure to traumatic material in the agency's attempts to understand what "went wrong;" the reviews of the events leading up to the death have been described as time consuming and are often critical of the workers' practice techniques (Regehr et al., 2002). Workers report being angry and frustrated with the review procedures and "red tape" that accompany a CMF (Cooper, 2005). In my own study of CWWs, similar sentiments were noted, even though some of these sentiments were outliers from the majority of the workers in my sample.

- "In a way a review of a case is necessary but not to pinpoint the downfalls of the worker because the worker has already done that. Reviewers are so focused on the worker's flaws and mistakes that they forget about the murderer."
- "Less finger pointing by the state agency involved. We get enough of that from the media and from the community. Stop trying to find out 'what we did wrong.' ... I realize that there is a need to study the case and understand where we could have done a better job for this child, but not at the expense of making the workers feel that they are the cause of the death."
- "I feel the worker should have the chance to speak to child fatality review board with out [sic] supervisors involved and without fear of retaliation. Rarely, in my career, has a child died when the front line social worker was not actively verbalizing [sic] concerns to supervision. We can only help as much as we are allowed by direct supervision, when a fatality occurs, we must remain silent...or lose our jobs and nothing is learned from the event."

The impact of a child's death and the agency's response is more than just an academic exercise, there is evidence that when workers experience a "critical event" while on the job, that it may have an impact on their current job performance, which is the primary reason that I include this information in the current chapter.

4.3.1 Post-Traumatic Stress and Child Welfare

An individual who has post-traumatic stress (PTS) has experienced a traumatic event, such as an accident, war, or victimization, and then experiences psychological distress related to this event: distressing recollections, thoughts, and dreams about the event or feeling as if the traumatic event were reoccurring again. In the most serious of cases, individuals meeting specific criteria and a clinical cut-off are diagnosed with post-traumatic stress disorder (PTSD) (American Psychiatric Association, 2000). Since the 1990s, a growing body of literature has explored the relationship between the traumatic experiences to which CWWs are exposed and later mental health concerns, including PTS and burnout (Bride, Jones, & MacMaster, 2007; Horwitz, 1998, 2006; Perron & Hiltz, 2006). The literature reports higher rates of PTS among social workers than among the general population. Specifically, in a single year, 15.2% of social workers meet the criteria for PTSD (Bride, 2007), compared to 3.5% of the general population (Kessler, Chiu, Demler, & Walters, 2005). Further, research has also found that CWWs have higher rates of psychological distress than among the general population (Cornille & Meyers, 1999).

Research shows that experiencing a major trauma can overwhelm one's capacities and have a negative effect on daily functioning, as well as mental and physical well-being (Fullilove et al., 1993; Herman, 1992; Resnick, Kilpatrick, Dansky, Saunders, & Best, 1993). PTS symptoms can serve as an impediment to the field of child welfare and social work. CWWs with higher levels of PTS symptoms are more likely to experience burnout, professional fatigue (Dane, 2000; Van Hook & Rothenberg, 2009), and disengagement from professional responsibilities (Perron & Hiltz, 2006), which places their clients at risk for not receiving optimum levels of treatment and services. Thus, the after-effects of workplace trauma can have important implications for children and families who are already involved in the child welfare system; workers struggling with a response to trauma and burn-out may be less effective at his or her job (Horwitz, 1998).

4.3.2 Workers' Response to Experiencing a CMF

Despite all of the work that had been done on CWWs' exposure to trauma and resulting PTS, there's been very little written about how maltreatment fatalities may play a role in this area. In my study of CWWs, those who experienced a CMF described reactions and emotions that are similar to PTS (Douglas, 2013). Of those who had a child on their caseload die, almost two-thirds of the respondents indicated that the bureaucratic process that followed the death of the child was a source of stress for them. Others described it having an impact on their professional and personal lives.

- "Difficulty sleeping, more emotional, trial of abuser was stressful, asked not to be assigned to as many infant/ young children cases, became even harder once I became pregnant and had my own child, I left protective services …to do juvenile delinquency work because the children were older and less vulnerable."
- "I was very stressed and I started questioning myself on every case. I had a hard time focusing on my other cases after the fatality."
- "I am very protective of my own children. I can't or don't leave them with anyone else or have a hard time keeping my one year old at a daycare setting."
- "I realized that I am numb to events such as this, but I still felt disappointed in my agency for not protecting better."
- "It certainly made me more paranoid about the possibility of it happening again."

The prevalence of CWWs in my study who met the criteria for PTSD (Andrykowski, Cordova, Studts, & Miller, 1998) was higher than among the general population, which was not surprising. Nationwide, 3.5% of the population meet the criteria for PTSD in a single year (Kessler et al., 2005); 12.5% of the workers in this study met the criteria for PTSD. Using the literature on trauma as a base (Fullilove et al., 1993; Herman, 1992; Resnick et al., 1993), I hypothesized that workers who experienced a CMF would have higher rates of PTS, which turned out to be inaccurate. The percent of workers who had experienced a CMF and met the criteria for PTSD was higher at 15%, compared with 12% who had not experienced a fatality. But that difference was not large enough to be of any statistical significance.

Next I considered only workers who had experienced a CMF on their caseload. In other words, I excluded all of the workers who did not experience the death of a child client. I examined whether workers' perceptions around the handling of the case were related to whether they had more PTS responses and found that they were. Workers who believed that the child's death was unavoidable had lower rates of PTS symptoms. This finding suggests that if workers' believe that the death of the child was out of their hands then the event is less traumatic for them. On the other hand, workers who reported that they were closely monitoring the family when the child died had overall higher rates of PTS symptoms. Both of these findings are similar to previous research on CWWs which found that workers who feel that they cannot do enough for their clients have higher levels of trauma symptoms (Horwitz, 2006). In a nutshell, workers who feel responsible for the traumatic events that their clients experience are more likely to experience mental distress and may be in need of assessment, support, intervention, or treatment. The way that a child's death is handled internally or by the media may potentially play a role in the level of responsibility that a worker feels. These findings could shape agency responses to children's deaths. Finally, the only measure that I included to assess the aftermath of a CMF was PTS. There are many other ways that a CMF might affect a worker, such as through other types of mental health concerns, stress responses, or impaired work performance and judgment that I did not investigate, but would be important for future research.

4.3.3 Supporting Workers After a CMF

"The lack of support from the management made the whole experience horrible both professionally and personal. 6 years later I still feel like I'm not always treated fairly because of the situation."

This is a quote from a worker who experienced the death of a child on her caseload. The literature on what promotes resilience among the general public and also populations that have experienced trauma points to the importance of having supportive relationships as a way to promote positive outcomes (Garmezy, 1993; Horwitz, 1998; Wyman, Cowen, Work, Work, & Parker 1991). This has been examined among CWWs, too. In fact, the research shows that having support from one's work peers is negatively related to PTS symptoms—when workers feel positively supported by their peers they are less likely to experience symptoms of PTS (Bride et al., 2007). One way to promote resilience and positive outcomes among CWWs is to build agency-based supports which encourage or enable workers to confide in a trusted individual or co-worker (Dane, 2000). Further, the literature on how fatalities have an impact on the workplace has discussed how to adequately support workers who have experienced a CMF through appropriate supervision (Gustavsson & MacEachron, 2002, 2004) and critical incident debriefing (Horwath, 1995; Weuste, 2006). Critical incident debriefing is a form of short-term, focused psychotherapy that offers support around a specific, immediate event that is often related to incidents in the workplace (Bisson, McFarlane, & Rose, 2000). In addition to what has been recommended in the literature, CWWs have reported their desire to receive more support from administrators and less "red tape" as a way to better manage their professional responsibilities (Van Hook & Rothenberg, 2009).

4.3.4 Support Provided After Fatality

I examined how many of the CWWs in my study had received formal support from their agencies. I found that less than half of workers reported that their agencies provided them with therapy/support after the fatality. This lack of formal support is surprising given the growing attention to "critical incidents" in the workplace (Attridge & VandePol, 2010; Declercq, Meganck, Deheeger, & Van Hoorde, 2011), secondary trauma among child welfare professionals (Bride et al., 2007; Dane, 2000; Horwitz, 2006), and the widespread movement to provide grief counseling when the death of a community member is unexpected (Thompson, 1995; Wenckstern & Leenaars, 1993). Formal support was offered to supervisors one-and-a-half times as often as it was to frontline workers. This may be because it is assumed that supervisors will provide support for frontline staff and thus, supervisors need a different level of support. Of those who reported that therapy was available, just over half used this service. The vast majority of those individuals assessed it as helpful. Nevertheless, when I compared those who received psychotherapy with those that did not, there was no difference in their levels of PTS symptoms, suggesting that even though it may have been helpful, there was no measurable difference in terms of mental health distress.

Most CWWs who experience the death of a child get support right where they work. Between 68 and 80% of workers reported that their co-workers and supervisors were a source of support for them, which is consistent with previous research concerning coping with the death of a child client (Regehr et al., 2002). The level of support that workers received was also not related to how many PTS symptoms they experienced. Even though workers may have relied on colleagues and found this helpful, that help did not yield positive gains in terms PTS symptoms. When asked what would help workers manage the difficult aftermath of fatality, workers volunteered many suggestions: additional emotional and legal support from their agencies, agency-funded counseling, and guidance regarding being sued and other matters that might arise during a trial that follows a CMF. The results of the study that I conducted were clear: In the aftermath of a fatality, workers do not feel supported and want more support from their agencies. The following are examples of workers' responses when asked how agencies could better support workers who experience a CMF.

- "Be supportive and not look for someone to blame. Often there were several people involved with the child before the incident. We need to be helpful and help our fellow workers through the tough times."
- "Create employment policies/programs that automatically engage the professional in a therapeutic way as the professional in this situation will often be unaware of the impact it has had on them until much later."
- "An agency should address all workers, foster parents, as well as the family who have experienced this loss. Services to provide support after the fatality should be mandatory, and NEVER should this just be one team, or workers [sic] job to handle all of the 'child fatalities!!!'"

4.4 The Bottom Line

The bottom line about the intersection of the child welfare profession and maltreatment fatalities is that despite all of the press coverage and attention to CMFs that occur under the watchful eye of child protection services, we know little about this part of the child welfare profession. Most of the research in this one area comes from the one study that I conducted on 426 CWWs in 2010–2011. This is an area demanding future attention and research.

4.4.1 What We Know

This is an under-researched area, but we can safely conclude the following.

- CWWs appear to be woefully prepared to recognize risk factors for maltreatment fatalities. At a bare minimum, workers should know that most deaths result from neglect, that most children die in the care of their mothers, and that about half of children who die from maltreatment are under the age of 1. Workers' knowledge on the latter characteristic is very good; there needs to be drastic improvement on the other two and many additional risk factors.
- On average, workers who experience the death of a child do not appear to be young or inexperienced. Workers are in middle adulthood, have about 6 years work experience, and have adequate education do be doing child welfare work.
- Experiencing a fatality on one's caseload does not appear to be related to experiencing PTS symptoms. Nevertheless, individual comments by workers suggest that they do not feel adequately supported in the aftermath of a child's death and less than half were offered formal sources of support, such as psychotherapy.

4.4 The Bottom Line

4.4.2 What Remains Unknown

In many respects, the research field is wide open in the area of CMFs. The one study that I conducted on the child welfare profession and fatalities should be replicated to confirm the findings. The field could benefit from addressing some additional questions:

- Where do workers get their information about maltreatment fatalities?
- How do workers respond to high-risk situations, such as a parent indicating that he or she might kill a child? Are these responses related to training, education, years on the job, etc.?

We know almost nothing about the pathway of child welfare practice that might end in a CMF. There are many questions to be addressed here, but one of the most pressing might be: Does focusing on family strengths distract CWWs from assessing for risk for maltreatment and potential fatality?

- How do attitudes about fatalities inform how workers practice child welfare work?
- Does experiencing a CMF on one's caseload impair a worker in ways for which I did not assess—such as other mental health concerns, stress responses, or impaired professional judgment and work performance.

This is a chapter that doesn't have a lot of good news about the child welfare profession and CMFs. During my testimony to the U.S. National Commission to Eliminate Child Abuse & Neglect Fatalities, I was asked if child welfare practice and its outcomes are "better than a coin toss." I believe that they are. Over the past three decades, there have been increases in federal legislation, new research, and new practice techniques to guide the profession. I do believe that hundreds or thousands of children's deaths are prevented annually, because of child welfare interventions, but we have no measure for tracking that and these kinds of stories remain hidden from the media because of confidentiality clauses. That said, I don't know if these deaths are prevented because of calculated child welfare practice techniques or because of luck—or a combination of the two. The bright light in this area is that the child welfare profession is poised and ready to take action in order to more effectively meet the needs of their clients. Additionally, there is a plethora of research being conducted by academics and researchers at private research firms and government agencies. I am hopeful that this research will increasingly turn its attention to help the field better understand how and when the child welfare profession intersects with the deaths of children who fall victim to abuse or neglect and how CWWs can help to prevent more children's deaths.

References

ACTION for Child Protection. (2010). *Assessing caregiver protective capacities related to parenting*. Retrieved January 3, 2015, from http://action4cp.org/documents/2010/pdf/June_2010_Assessing_Caregiver_Protective_Capacities.pdf

American Psychiatric Association. (2000). *Diagnostic and statistical manual of mental health disorders* (Revised 4th ed.). Washington, DC: Author.

American Psychological Association. (2013). Guidelines for psychological evaluation in child protection matters. *American Psychologist, 68*(1), 20–31.

Anderson, R., Ambrosino, R., Valentine, D., & Lauderdale, M. (1983). Child deaths attributed to abuse and neglect: An empirical study. *Children and Youth Services Review, 5*(1), 75–89.

Andrykowski, M. A., Cordova, M. J., Studts, J. L., & Miller, T. W. (1998). Posttraumatic stress disorder after treatment for breast cancer: Prevalence of diagnosis and use of the PTSD Checklist – Civilian Version (PCL–C) as a screening instrument. *Journal of Consulting and Clinical Psychology, 66*, 586–590.

Antle, B. F., Frey, S. E., Sar, B. K., Barbee, A. P., & van Zyl, M. A. (2009). Training the child welfare workforce in healthy couple relationships: An examination of attitudes and outcomes. *Children and Youth Services Review, 32*(2), 223–230.

Arad-Davidzon, B., & Benbenishty, R. (2008). The role of workers' attitudes and parent and child wishes in child protection workers' assessments and recommendation regarding removal and reunification. *Children and Youth Services Review, 30*(1), 107–121.

Attridge, M., & VandePol, B. (2010). The business case for workplace critical incident response: A literature review and some employer examples. *Journal of Workplace Behavioral Health, 25*(2), 132–145.

Ayre, P. (2001). Child protection and the media: Lessons from the last three decades. *British Journal of Social Work, 31*(6), 887–901.

Baber, K., & Bean, G. (2009). Frameworks: A community-based approach to preventing youth suicide. *Journal of Community Psychology, 37*(6), 684–696.

Barth, R. P., Lloyd, E. C., Christ, S. L., Chapman, M. V., & Dickinson, N. S. (2008). Child welfare worker characteristics and job satisfaction: A national study. *Social Work, 53*(3), 199–209.

Batty, D. (2001, September 28). Inexperienced social worker left to make complex decisions. *The Guardian*. Retrieved from http://www.guardian.co.uk/society/2001/sep/28/2

Baumann, D., Law, J. R., Sheets, J., Reid, G., & Graham, J. C. (2005). Evaluating the effectiveness of actuarial risk assessment models. *Children and Youth Services Review, 27*(5), 465–490.

Beveridge, J. (1994). Analysis of Colorado child maltreatment fatalities. *Colorado's Children, 13*(2), 3–6.

Bisson, J. I., McFarlane, A. C., & Rose, S. (2000). Psychological debriefing. In E. B. Foa, T. M. Keane, & M. J. Friedman (Eds.), *Effective treatments for PTSD: Practice guidelines from the International Society for Traumatic Stress Studies* (pp. 39–59). New York, NY: Guilford Press.

Bride, B. E. (2007). Prevalence of secondary traumatic stress among social workers. *Social Work, 52*(1), 63–70.

Bride, B. E., Jones, J. L., & MacMaster, S. A. (2007). Correlates of secondary traumatic stress in child protective services workers. *Journal of Evidence-Based Social Work, 4*(3/4), 69–80. doi:10.1300/J394v04n03_05.

Brun, C., & Rapp, R. C. (2001). Strengths-based case management: Individuals' perspectives on strengths and the case manager relationship. *Social Work, 46*(3), 278–288.

Budd, K. S. (2005). Assessing parenting capacity in a child welfare context. *Children and Youth Services Review, 27*(4), 429–444. doi:http://dx.doi.org/10.1016/j.childyouth.2004.11.008.

Bundy-Fazioli, K., Briar-Lawson, K., & Hardiman, E. R. (2009). A qualitative examination of power between child welfare workers and parents. *British Journal of Social Work, 39*(8), 1447–1464. doi:10.1093/bjsw/bcn038.

Camasso, M. J., & Jagannathan, R. (1995). Prediction accuracy of the Washington and Illinois risk assessment instruments: An application of receiver operating characteristic curve analysis. *Social Work Research, 19*(3), 174–183.

Chance, T. C., & Scannapieco, M. (2002). Ecological correlates of child maltreatment: Similarities and differences between child fatality and nonfatality cases. *Child and Adolescent Social Work Journal, 19*(2), 139–161.

Child Welfare League of America, I. (1999). *Child welfare standards of excellence.* Washington, DC: Child Welfare League of America, Inc.

Collins, M. E., Amodeo, M., & Clay, C. (2008). Planning and evaluating child welfare training projects: Working toward a comprehensive conceptual model. *Child Welfare, 87*(5), 69–86.

Cooper, L. (2005). Implications of media scrutiny for a child protection agency. *Journal of Sociology and Social Welfare, 32*(3), 107–121.

Cordero, L., Rudd, M. D., Bryan, C. J., & Corso, K. A. (2008). Accuracy of primary care medical providers' understanding of the FDA black box warning label for antidepressants. *Primary Care & Community Psychiatry, 13*(3), 109–114.

Cornille, T. A., & Meyers, T. W. (1999). Secondary traumatic stress among child protective service workers. *Traumatology, 5*(1), 15–31. doi:10.1177/153476569900500105.

County of Los Angeles Children's Special Investigation Unit. (2012). *2011 Recurring systemic issues report.* Los Angeles, CA: Department of Children and Family Services.

Csikai, E. L., Herrin, C., Tang, M., & Church Ii, W. T. (2008). Serious illness, injury, and death in child protection and preparation for end-of-life situations among child welfare services workers. *Child Welfare, 87*(6), 49–70.

Curry, D., McCarragher, T., & Dellmann-Jenkins, M. (2005). Training, transfer, and turnover: Exploring the relationship among transfer of learning factors and staff retention in child welfare. *Children and Youth Services Review, 27*(8), 931–948.

D'Andrade, A., Austin, M. J., & Benton, A. (2008). Risk and safety assessment in child welfare: Instrument comparisons. *Journal of Evidence-Based Social Work, 5*(1/2), 31–56. doi:10.1300/J394v05n01-03.

Damashek, A., Nelson, M. M., & Bonner, B. L. (2013). Fatal child maltreatment: Characteristics of deaths from physical abuse versus neglect. *Child Abuse & Neglect, 37*(10), 735–744. doi:http://dx.doi.org/10.1016/j.chiabu.2013.04.014.

Dane, B. (2000). Child welfare workers: An innovative approach for interacting with secondary trauma. *Journal of Social Work Education, 36*(1), 27–38.

Davidson-Arad, B., & Benbenishty, R. (2010). Contribution of child protection workers' attitudes to their risk assessments and intervention recommendations: A study in Israel. *Health & Social Care in the Community, 18*(1), 1–9. doi:10.1111/j.1365-2524.2009.00868.x.

Declercq, F. d. r., Meganck, R., Deheegher, J., & Van Hoorde, H. (2011). Frequency of and subjective response to critical incidents in the prediction of PTSD in emergency personnel. *Journal of Traumatic Stress, 24*(1), 133–136.

Douglas, E. M. (2009). Media coverage of agency-related child maltreatment fatalities: Does it result in state legislative change intended to prevent future fatalities? *Journal of Policy Practice, 8*(3), 224–239.

Douglas, E. M. (2012). Child welfare workers' training, knowledge, and practice concerns regarding child maltreatment fatalities: An exploratory, multi-state analysis. *Journal of Public Child Welfare, 6*(5), 659–677. doi:10.1080/15548732.2012.723975.

Douglas, E. M. (2013). Symptoms of posttraumatic stress among child welfare workers who experience a maltreatment fatality on their caseload. *Journal of Evidence-Based Social Work, 10*(4), 373–387. doi:10.1080/15433714.2012.664058.

Douglas, E. M., Mohn, B. L., & Gushwa, M. (2015). The presence of maltreatment fatality-related content in pre-service child welfare training curricula: A brief report of 20 states. *Child & Adolescent Social Work Journal, 32*(3), 213–218.

Douglas, E. M., & Serino, P. J. (2013). The extent of evidence-based information about child maltreatment fatalities in social science textbooks. *Journal of Evidence-Based Social Work, 10*(5), 447–454. doi:10.1080/15433714.2012.759839.

English, D. J., & Pecora, P. J. (1994). Risk assessment as a practice method in child protective services. *Child Welfare, 73*(5), 451–473.

Franke, T., Bagdasaryan, S., & Furman, W. (2009). A multivariate analysis of training, education, and readiness for public child welfare practice. *Children and Youth Services Review, 31*(12), 1330–1336.

Fullilove, M. T., Fullilove Iii, R. E., Smith, M., Winkler, K., Michael, C., Panzer, P. G., et al. (1993). Violence, trauma, and post-traumatic stress disorder among women drug users. *Journal of Traumatic Stress, 6*(4), 533–543.

Gainsborough, J. (2009). Scandals, lawsuits, and politics: Child welfare policy in the United States. *State Politics & Policy Quarterly, 9*(3), 325–355.

Garmezy, N. (1993). Children in poverty: Resilience despite risk. *Psychiatry, 56*(1), 127–136.

Gelles, R. J. (1996). *The book of David: How preserving families can cost children's lives.* New York, NY: Basic Books.

Gelles, R. J. (2003). *Failure to protect: Interview – Richard Gelles.* Retrieved from http://www.pbs.org/wgbh/pages/frontline/shows/fostercare/inside/gelles.html

Graham, J. C., Stepura, K., Baumann, D. J., & Kern, H. (2010). Predicting child fatalities among less-severe CPS investigations. *Children and Youth Services Review, 32*(2), 274–280.

Graybeal, C. (2001). Strengths-based social work assessment: Transforming the dominant paradigm. *Families in Society, 82*(3), 233–242.

Gustavsson, N., & MacEachron, A. E. (2002). Death and the child welfare worker. *Children and Youth Services Review, 24*(12), 903–915.

Gustavsson, N., & MacEachron, A. E. (2004). When a child welfare client dies: An agency-centered perspective. *Child Welfare: Journal of Policy, Practice, and Program, 83*(4), 317–340.

Herman, J. L. (1992). Complex PTSD: A syndrome in survivors of prolonged and repeated trauma. *Journal of Traumatic Stress, 5*(3), 377–391.

Horwath, J. (1995). The impact of fatal child abuse cases on staff: Lessons for trainers and managers. *Child Abuse Review, 4*(Special Issue), 351–355.

Horwitz, M. (1998). Social worker trauma: Building resilience in child protection social workers. *Smith College Studies in Social Work, 68*(3), 363–377.

Horwitz, M. J. (2006). Work-related trauma effects in child protection social workers. *Journal of Social Service Research, 32*(3), 1–18.

Huebner, R. A., Jones, B. L., Miller, V. P., Custer, M., & Critchfield, B. (2006). Comprehensive family services and customer satisfaction outcomes. *Child Welfare: Journal of Policy, Practice, and Program, 85*(4), 691–714.

Jones, L. P., & Okamura, A. (2000). Reprofessionalizing child welfare services: An evaluation of a Title IVE training program. *Research on Social Work Practice, 10*(5), 607–621.

Kemp, S. P., Marcenko, M. O., Lyons, S. J., & Kruzich, J. M. (2014). Strength-based practice and parental engagement in child welfare services: An empirical examination. *Children and Youth Services Review, 47*, 27–35. doi:10.1016/j.childyouth.2013.11.001.

Kessler, R. C., Chiu, W. T., Demler, O., & Walters, E. E. (2005). Prevalence, severity, and comorbidity of 12-month DSM-IV disorders in the National Comorbidity Survey Replication. *Archives of General Psychiatry, 62*(6), 617–627. doi:10.1001/archpsyc.62.6.617.

Keys, M. (2009). Determining the skills for child protection practice: From quandary to quagmire? *Child Abuse Review, 18*(5), 297–315.

Lachman, P., & Bernard, C. (2006). Moving from blame to quality: How to respond to failures in child protective services. *Child Abuse & Neglect, 30*(9), 963–968.

Levenson, M. (2015). DCF's new strategy could see more families split up. *Boston Globe.* Retrieved from https://www.bostonglobe.com/metro/2015/10/11/conflict-inherent-dcf-mission-statement/hKkPNJ8tto1xp01yuHzP4I/story.html

Lietz, C. A. (2011). Theoretical adherence to family centered practice: Are strengths-based principles illustrated in families' descriptions of child welfare services? *Children and Youth Services Review, 33*(6), 888–893. doi:10.1016/j.childyouth.2010.12.012.

Lietz, C. A., & Rounds, T. (2009). Strengths-based supervision: A child welfare supervision training project. *Clinical Supervisor, 28*(2), 124–140. doi:10.1080/07325220903334065.

References

Mapp, S. C. (2002). A framework for family visiting for children in long-term foster care. *Families in Society, 83*(2), 175–182.

Moon, R. Y., Weese-Mayer, D. E., & Silvestri, J. M. (2003). Nighttime child care: Inadequate sudden infant death syndrome risk factor knowledge, practice, and policies. *Pediatrics, 111*(4), 795.

Murphy, P. (1997). *Wasted: The plight of America's unwanted children*. Chicago, IL: Ivan R. Dee Publisher.

National Coalition for Child Protection Reform. (2009). The real reasons for child abuse deaths. *Issue Paper, 8*, from http://www.nccpr.org/reports/8Realreasons.pdf

Ojofeitimi, E. O., Asekun-Olarinmoye, E. O., Bamidele, J. O., Owolabi, O. O., Oladele, E. A., & Orji, E. O. (2009). Poor knowledge of causes and prevention of stillbirths among health care providers. *International Journal of Childbirth Education, 24*(4), 26–29.

Perron, B., & Hiltz, B. (2006). Burnout and secondary trauma among forensic interviewers of abused children. *Child & Adolescent Social Work Journal, 23*(2), 216–234. doi:10.1007/s10560-005-0044-3.

Probst, B. (2010). Implicit and explicit use of the strengths perspective in social work education. *Journal of Teaching in Social Work, 30*(4), 468–484.

Rapp, C. A., Saleebey, D., & Sullivan, W. P. (2005). The future of strengths-based social work. *Advances in Social Work, 6*(1), 79–90.

Regehr, C., Bogo, M., Shlonsky, A., & LeBlanc, V. (2010). Confidence and professional judgment in assessing children's risk of abuse. *Research on Social Work Practice, 20*(6), 621–628. doi:10.1177/1049731510368050.

Regehr, C., Chau, S., Leslie, B., & Howe, P. (2002). Inquiries into deaths of children in care: The impact on child welfare workers and their organization. *Children and Youth Services Review, 24*(12), 885–902.

Resnick, H. S., Kilpatrick, D. G., Dansky, B. S., Saunders, B. E., & Best, C. L. (1993). Prevalence of civilian trauma and posttraumatic stress disorder in a representative national sample of women. *Journal of Consulting and Clinical Psychology, 61*(6), 984–991. doi:10.1037/0022-006x.61.6.984.

Saleebey, D. (1992). *The strengths perspective in social work practice*. New York, NY: Longman.

Saleebey, D. (1996). The strengths perspective in social work practice: Extensions and cautions. *Social Work, 41*(3), 296–305.

Saleebey, D. (2009). Introduction: Power in the people. In D. Saleebey (Ed.), *The strengths perspective in social work practice* (5th ed., pp. 1–23). New York, NY: Pearson Education, Inc.

Scharfenberg, D., & Miller, J. (2015, September 28). Revamped DCF policies will put kids first, governor says. *Boston Globe*. Retrieved from https://www.bostonglobe.com/metro/2015/09/28/baker-discuss-changes-department-children-and-families-state-house/bSIb2IbgApV2khJLFd41iM/story.html

Sheely, A. I., & Bratton, S. C. (2010). A strengths-based parenting intervention with low-income African American families. *Professional School Counseling, 13*(3), 175–183.

Shlonsky, A., & Wagner, D. (2005). The next step: Integrating actuarial risk assessment and clinical judgment into an evidence-based practice framework in CPS case management. *Children and Youth Services Review, 27*(4), 409–427. doi:10.1016/j.childyouth.2004.11.007.

Siegal, H. A., Rapp, R. C., Kelliher, C. W., & Fisher, J. H. (1995). The strengths perspective of case management: A promising inpatient substance abuse treatment enhancement. *Journal of Psychoactive Drugs, 27*(1), 67–72.

Smith, B. D. (2008). Child welfare service plan compliance: Perceptions of parents and caseworkers. *Families in Society, 89*(4), 521–532.

Staudt, M., Howard, M. O., & Drake, B. (2001). The operationalization, implementation, and effectiveness of the strengths perspective: A review of empirical studies. *Journal of Social Service Research, 27*(3), 1–21.

Strand, V. C., & Bosco-Ruggiero, S. (2010). Initiating and sustaining a mentoring program for child welfare staff. *Administration in Social Work, 34*(1), 49–67.

Thompson, R. A. (1995). Being prepared for suicide or sudden death in schools: Strategies to restore equilibrium. *Journal of Mental Health Counseling, 17*(3), 264–277.

U.S. Department of Health & Human Services. (2013). *Child maltreatment 2012: Reports from the States to the National Child Abuse and Neglect Data Systems – National statistics on child abuse and neglect.* Washington, DC: Administration for Children & Families, U.S. Department of Health & Human Services.

Van Hook, M. P., & Rothenberg, M. (2009). Quality of life and compassion satisfaction/fatigue and burnout in child welfare workers: A study of the child welfare workers in community based care organizations in Central Florida. *Social Work & Christianity, 36*(1), 36–54.

Weick, A. (2009). Issues in overturning a medical model of social work practice. *Reflections (10800220), 15*(3), 7–11.

Wenckstern, S., & Leenaars, A. A. (1993). Trauma and suicide in our schools. *Death Studies, 17*(2), 151–171.

Werrbach, G. B. (1996). Family-strengths-based intensive child case management. *Families in Society: The Journal of Contemporary Social Services, 77*(4), 216–226.

Weuste, M. B. (2006). *Critical incident stress and debriefing of child welfare workers.* 66, ProQuest Information & Learning, US. Retrieved from http://search.ebscohost.com/login.aspx?direct=true&db=psyh&AN=2006-99001-024&site=ehost-live

Wyman, P. A., Cowen, E. L., Work, W. C., Work, W. C., & Parker, G. R. (1991). Developmental and family milieu correlates of resilience in urban children who have experienced major life stress. *American Journal of Community Psychology, 19*(3), 405–426.

Chapter 5
Child Death Review Teams

The current chapter builds on the previous by exploring the policies and programs that have been put in place to better identify and ultimately prevent child maltreatment fatalities (CMFs). This chapter focuses on child death review teams[1] (CDRTs), their history and purpose, the work that they complete, and how that work relates to changes in policy and practice in the response to and prevention of CMFs. Like the chapters that came before, this chapter will also highlight the controversies surrounding and areas of disagreement or limitations of CDRTs.

- It is generally understood that CDRTs focus on prevention. That said, members of the legal and criminal justice professions are well represented on CDRTs, even though they do not generally work on prevention.
- There is limited research on the outputs of CDRTs, making it difficult to understand the scope of their work.
- Relatedly, there is limited research on the effectiveness of CDRTs To date there has been no systematic review of the effectiveness of the CDRT movement and whether fewer children die as a result of this work.

5.1 Child Death Review Teams

CDRTs are multidisciplinary workgroups that review deaths of children in order to identify opportunities for prevention and intervention. When CMFs first caught public attention in the United States, one of the earliest organized efforts in response to these events was the development of review teams—professionals that review the cases of deceased children in an effort to identify problems that may have led or

---

[1] The terms "Child death review" and "child fatality review" are used interchangeably, as are "teams" and "panels" to refer to this multidisciplinary workgroup. I primary use the term child death review, CDR, or child death review team, CDRT, in this book, but may occasionally use alternate language in order to be consistent with the literature or other resources.

contributed to the death. The first CDRT was established in 1978 in Los Angeles County, California. CDRTs perform multidisciplinary, multi-agency reviews of child fatalities in a given county, district, or state (Gellert, Maxwell, Durfee, & Wagner, 1995). Today there are two national centers that provide guidance concerning child death review in the U.S., the National Center for the Review and Prevention of Child Deaths (http://www.childdeathreview.org/) and the National Center on Child Fatality Review (http://ican4kids.org/ncfr_History.asp).

According to the National Center for the Review and Prevention of Child Deaths, all states in the United States, plus the nation's capital of the District of Columbia, have a CDRT; the majority of states have CDR legislation or an executive order mandating and/or providing guidance on child death review in their respective states; most of this legislation was passed between 1990 and 2000 (National Center for the Review and Prevention of Child Deaths, n.d.-b). The staff that CDRTs employ ranges from 0 to 4.75 full-time employees, with an average of about one full-time staff member. The budget for CDRTs ranges from $0 to $921,200, with a median annual budget of $90,000. In the beginning, CDRT activities were largely unfunded; today funding mechanisms include federal block grants, the Child Abuse Prevention & Treatment Act, the Children's Justice Act, state funding, and other creative sources of funding, such as in Arizona where they charge $1 on all requests for death certificates (National Center for the Review and Prevention of Child Deaths, 2010).

In the United States there is great variation concerning the nature of deaths that are reviewed; some states focus on all causes of death, such as natural, accidental, maltreatment, vehicular, suicide, etc., with others focusing exclusively on maltreatment-related deaths (American Academy of Pediatrics, 2010). This chapter focuses primarily on CDRT activities that concern fatal child maltreatment.

5.2 Purpose and Composition of CDRTs

CDRTs generally focused on prevention, investigation of a crime, or a combination of both. A study from the early 2000s interviewed CDRT leaders about a variety of characteristics concerning their state's teams (Webster, Schnitzer, Jenny, Ewigman, & Alario, 2003). The results showed that the majority of CDRTs focus on identifying the circumstances that led to a child's death, providing suggestions for the prevention of future child deaths, reviewing agency involvement and actions surrounding a child's death, and collecting data about child deaths for analysis at a later time. Just over a quarter of teams stated that they assist in the prosecution of fatal child maltreatment. A colleague and I reviewed 46 state statutes that provide guidance or mandates concerning the focus, composition, and activities of CDRTs (Douglas & McCarthy, 2011). With some modification, we based our analyses on the same categories as the earlier study by Webster and her colleagues and found similar results, displayed in Table 5.1. We found that the responses that team leaders gave in the early 2000s concerning the focus of CDRTs were consistent with the

5.2 Purpose and Composition of CDRTs

Table 5.1 Purpose of Child Death Review Teams by Source of Information

Purpose of CDRT	CDRT Representative (Webster et al., 2003)	CDRT State Statute (Douglas and McCarthy 2011)
Provide suggestions for the prevention of future child deaths	94%	89%
Identify circumstances leading to cause of death	94%	80%
Collect data about child deaths for later analysis	78%	77%
Review agency involvement and actions surrounding death	80%	57%
Provide suggestions for investigation of future child deaths	Was not asked	36%
Assist in prosecution of child maltreatment fatalities	27%	14%

Adapted from: Webster et al. (2003). Child death review: The state of the nation. *American Journal of Prevention medicine, 25*(5): 58–64 and Douglas and McCarthy (2011). Child death review teams: A content analysis of social policy. *Child Welfare, 90*(3): 91–110

focus as directed by state statute. The two areas of disagreement concerned reviewing agency involvement and actions surrounding the death and assisting in the prosecution of CMFs. In both instances, team leaders reported more involvement in these areas than was guided by statute.

As multidisciplinary workgroups, it is common for U.S. CDRTs to be comprised of representatives from the legal, child welfare, medical, public health, and mental health professions. Thus, a comprehensive team might consist of one or several state police officers, assistant district or attorneys general, child welfare supervisors/managers, medical examiners, pediatricians, coroners, public health nurse supervisors, maternal-child health professionals, school officials, and mental health professionals who specialize in abusive and neglectful families. On the less comprehensive side, a CDRT might be comprised of a state police officer, an assistant attorney general, a child welfare supervisor/manager and a medical examiner. Depending on state population and the rate of child deaths, CDRTs in the United States often exist at the county, regional, and/or state levels.

In our review of the legislation which creates, funds, and provides guidance concerning CDRTs, my colleague and I also found that even though state statutes and the teams themselves may place a heavy emphasis on activities related to prevention, members of the legal or investigative professions—lawyers, law enforcement, and medical examiners—have a strong presence on CDRTs. For example, the top six professional groups that are mandated to be represented on CDRTs include a: (1) legal representative (such as a district attorney)—mandated in 93% of states, (2) child welfare professional—93%, (3) law enforcement—88%, (4) public health professional—83%, (5) medical examiner—81%, and (6) pediatrician—79%. Half of these professional groups (legal representative, law enforcement, and medical examiner) are more closely aligned with criminal investigations. Members of these professions generally deal with fatalities *after* they have occurred; they may be concerned about prevention, but do not normally play an active role in preventing CMFs. At the same time, professionals which might be more in a position to prevent fatal maltreatment are not as likely to be represented, such as a child advocate—mandated in 37% of states, maternal-child health professional—30% and legislators—mandated in 12% of states. Additionally, no states specify the need for a researcher with expertise in children and families sit on CDRTs.

This is not to say that a preventive versus an investigative focus are mutually exclusive. They are not. My colleague and I ranked states according to the language and priorities stipulated in their state policy. Of the top two states ranking highest in investigation, Georgia and Texas, one was also ranked highest for a focus on prevention (Texas). At the same time, we found that states with higher crime rates are more likely to rank higher in both investigation and prevention regulations and activities. In many ways this makes sense—it speaks to states trying to solve a problem through dual efforts: prevention and punishment. Further, we found that states which passed legislation later rather than earlier are less likely to focus as much on investigation, which speaks to a potentially shifting attitude in the focus of CDRTs.

5.3 Selection Criteria and the Review Process

States have a variety of ways of determining which cases come before CDRTs. Some states review all children's deaths in the entire county/state, others focus on all deaths from external causes, and still others review only those related to abuse and neglect (Covington & Johnston, 2011). As stated, because of the focus of this book, I primarily examine CDRTs as they relate to CMFs. The categories of death and selection criteria which would most likely bring CMFs before CDRTs are the following: all medical examiner cases, homicides, death by abuse or neglect, and families that were known to or working with child protective services. These selection criteria are used by the majority of cases in the United States (National Center for the Review and Prevention of Child Deaths, 2010). It should be noted also, that most states conduct reviews retrospectively, after cases have worked their way through the criminal justice system or internal reviews of relevant state agencies (Douglas & McCarthy, 2011; Webster et al., 2003).

In conducting a review of a CMF case, a team would request and then review past records from agencies or service providers that may have had contact with the victim or family before death (Durfee & Durfee, 1995; Durfee, Durfee, & West, 2002). What a team can request and review, however, may depend on its subpoena power, or its ability to legally command receipt of evidence and information (Webster et al., 2003). For example, a team might request past records from (1) child welfare services, (2) mental health services, (3) medical providers such as a pediatrician, family physician, medical clinic, or hospital, (4) school systems, (5) public health services, (6) law enforcement agencies, (7) court records, and (8) any other agency that worked with or conducted an evaluation of the family. Moreover, these records could be requested about the victim, surviving siblings, or any of the caregivers. In addition to a paper review, a team might request that some of the professionals who worked with the family be present at the review. A staff assistant to the CDRT then summarizes this information for the team; reviews of cases are conducted during a single meeting in the course of several hours. Teams meet monthly or several times throughout the year (Bunting & Reid, 2005; Durfee et al., 2002; Durfee & Durfee, 1995; Hochstadt, 2006).

Generally the purpose of having professionals who worked with the family at the meeting is not to place blame, but to better understand the family and the services it received. Based on problems identified in the review, the team makes a series of "findings" which generally identify how the larger professional community may have missed an opportunity to meet the needs of the victim. Most often, each finding is coupled with a recommendation concerning how a professional community, a legislative body, or a specific agency could adapt its practices to better anticipate, understand, and meet the needs of its most vulnerable victims. The findings and recommendations of these confidential reviews are de-identified, or edited to remove identifying information (e.g., names, birthdates, etc.), compiled and presented in aggregate in a report made accessible to the public on the websites of each state's or county's CDRT (Douglas, 2005; Durfee & Durfee, 1995; Durfee, Gellert, & Durfee, 1992).

5.4 Outputs of Child Death Review Teams

The most common output from CDRTs is recommendations, which are issued in annual or near- annual reports issued by the team. Based on my own calculations of what information was available on the website for the National Center for the Review and Prevention of Child Deaths, 60.6% of states published annual information for the years 2003–2012. These recommendations usually identify gaps in services, communication errors within and between professional groups, a change in agency or state policy, training and education for the public or certain professional groups, or new approaches that need to be taken. Text Box 5.1 provides examples of recommendations from CDRTs around the U.S.

Text Box 5.1 Examples of Recommendations from Child Death Review Teams

Texas, 2011 Report

- Study and report on the feasibility of developing and implementing an automated electronic system that would identify new births to parents whose parental rights have been terminated or who have had a child die of maltreatment. The system would need to automatically trigger a Child Protective Service referral to assess the living situation of the newborn and to provide support services as needed to the newborn in a high-risk environment (Texas Child Fatality Review Team, 2011, p. 31).

(continued)

> **Text Box 5.1** (continued)
>
> **Wisconsin, 2010 Report**
>
> - Nursing-based home visiting programs to prevent child abuse and neglect.
>   - Registered nurse as the provider
>   - Target low-income, single, young parents
>   - Consistent visiting promotes healthy relationships between providers and parents (Children's Health Alliance of Wisconsin, 2010, p. 41).
>
> **Utah, 2005–2007 Report**
>
> - Increase education of parents on where to turn for help if they feel they are likely to harm their child, (Utah Department of Health, 2010, p. 19).
>
> **Pennsylvania, 2013 Report**
>
> - Local teams continue to recommend education and the development of child death scene protocols for each county (Pennsylvania Bureau of Family Health, 2013, p. 49).

A colleague and I collected and reviewed recommendations from U.S. CDRTs that were issued between 2000 and 2007; of the 37 state-level reports that we reviewed, 29 issued recommendations that were specific to maltreatment (Douglas & Cunningham, 2008). In total we categorized 313 recommendations relevant to preventing CMFs into 11 different content areas that those 29 states addressed. Table 5.2 shows the content areas, ranked by the number of states that endorsed each area of recommendation.

By taking stock of the recommendations issued by CDRTs, one is able to gain a unique view of the primary concerns of professionals working "in the trenches" with fatal maltreatment. Without a doubt, professionals are most concerned about educating the public concerning risk factors for maltreatment and how to report maltreatment if it is suspected or identified. The next group of recommendations moves away from the public and into the agencies that work with maltreating families. These recommendations emphasize the need for better communication both within and between agencies, for example child welfare workers communicating when a case is transferred between workers, or domestic violence and child welfare professionals working in partnership when providing services for the same family. The third most frequently cited recommendation is in the area of criminal investigations on children's deaths. If death scenes are unknowingly dismissed as potential crime scenes, it becomes nearly impossible to accurately identify and prosecute cases of fatal maltreatment (see Chapters 2 and 6 for more discussion).

Recommendations from CDRTs have been the subject of concern, however. Many times recommendations are written to express a general sentiment, but lack the level of specificity that is needed in order to direct or inspire action or hold

Table 5.2 Content Areas for Recommendations Made by Child Death Review Teams, by Rank Order

Content Area	Number of States Endorsed[a]
Public education—risk factors for maltreatment or reporting of maltreatment	23
Agency communication—between or within agencies	17
Child death investigation—changes in protocol	15
Training for professionals—in a wide array of issues concerning treating or recognizing maltreatment	12
Child welfare system—improvements in service delivery, caseloads	10
Risk factors/assessment—comprehensive risk assessments for families	10
Child death review teams—changes in review protocol or funding	8
Mandated reporting—training and enforcement for mandated reporters	8
Home visiting programs—increase in programming	6
Criminal responsibility—increased penalties	5

[a]Out of n = 29
As reported in Douglas, E. M., & Cunningham, J. M. (2008). Recommendations from child fatality review teams: Results of a US nationwide exploratory study concerning maltreatment fatalities and social service delivery. *Child Abuse Review, 17*(5), 331–351. doi:10.1002/car.1044

groups or individuals accountable. This topic has been explored by Wirtz and colleagues (Wirtz, Foster, & Lenart, 2011) who lay out a template for drafting effective recommendations. These authors argue that in addition to accurately identifying the problem areas and activities currently underway to address the problem area, recommendations should specify: (1) who or what group will take action, (2) the intended recipient of the action, (3) how the action should be taken, (4) who will be held accountable for said action, (5) decision-makers or funders who will be notified of the need for action, and (6) the documentation/tracking of outcomes.

Wirtz and his colleagues scored 941 recommendations from 76 CDRT reports, on their level of effectiveness, from 1 to 5, with 1 being least effective; they determined that most recommendations have low to modest effectiveness, with mean scores ranging from 2 to 3. They found that CDRTs struggled most with articulating (1) who would be responsible for taking action, (2) addressing the issue of accountability, and (3) the documentation of outcomes. In Table 5.3, I provide examples of two actual, but less effective, recommendations that were made by CDRTs between 2010 and 2013. I then used the criteria provided by Wirtz and colleagues to show how they could be improved. I did not include the names of the states that made these recommendations in order to protect their identity.

5.5 Wide Acceptance and Use of Child Death Review Teams

Review teams have gained support and recognition from professionals, advocates, and decision-makers—as evidenced by their popularity throughout the United States, as well as other nations worldwide (Brandon, Dodsworth, & Rumball, 2005;

Table 5.3 Examples of Ineffective Recommendations from CDRT Reports

Example of Written Recommendation	Intervention—Actor: Who Will Act?	Intervention—Focus: Who is Recipient?	Specificity of Action: How to Proceed?	Accountability: Who will Track Progress?
Example 1				
Actual: Provide continuing education regarding death scene investigation	None stated	None stated	None stated	None stated
Better: The State Police should work with the National Center for the Prosecution of Child Abuse to increase detective's investigative skills for handling death scenes involving children. CDRT will provide training support and evaluate training.	The State Police	State Police detectives	Specific focus on implementing training with national center	CDRT
Example 2				
Actual: Continue statewide efforts to prevent abusive head trauma and other forms of child abuse.	None stated	None stated	None stated	None stated
Better: The Local Center for the Prevention of Shaken Baby Syndrome (LCPSBS) should work with the state association of hospitals/birthing centers to implement prevention programs to all parents of newborns re: SBS. Progress will be reported by LCPSBS.	Local Center for the Prevention of Shaken Baby Syndrome and State association of hospitals/birthing centers	Hospitals and birthing centers and parents of newborns	Specific focus on training regarding prevention of SBS	Local Center for the Prevention of Shaken Baby Syndrome

Adapted from Wirtz, et al. (2011). Assessing and improving child death review team recommendations. *Injury Prevention, 17,* 64–70

Bunting & Reid, 2005; Devaney, Lazenbatt, & Bunting, 2011; Durfee et al., 2002; Reder & Duncan, 1999; Vincent, 2010). As of 2009, in addition to the United States there were known CDR activities in Australia, Canada, England, Japan, Lebanon, the Philippines, Scotland, and Wales (Durfee, Parra, & Alexander, 2009). Further, the World Health Organization and some of their collaborators have written about and promoted the merits of CDR (Theiss-Nyland & Rechel, 2013). The work and activities of CDRTs have been most discussed by professionals in the United States (Covington, 2011; Durfee & Durfee, 1995; Durfee et al., 1992; Schnitzer, Covington, Wirtz, Verhoek-Oftedahl, & Palusci, 2008; Shanley, Risch, & Bonner, 2010; Webster et al., 2003) and England (Bunting & Reid, 2005; Mazzola, Mohiddin, Ward, & Holdsworth, 2013; Sidebotham, Fox, Horwath, & Powell, 2011; Ward Platt, 2014). Further, recent comparative studies on CDR at the international level have focused on differences and similarities in practice techniques (Axford & Bullock, 2005; Vincent, 2010).

There is a wide body of literature that discusses the merits of CDRTs and the opportunities for learning and change. The CDRT model provides a unique opportunity to review cases in-depth from multiple disciplines and plan for how one might act in the future, as has been recognized by members of the health professions (Berkowitz, 2008; Luallen et al., 1998). The part of the U.S. Department of Health & Human Services' "Healthy People 2020" initiative that focuses on family violence recommends that 90% of children's deaths due to external causes be reviewed by CDRTs (U.S. Department of Health & Human Services, n.d.). Further, the American Academy of Pediatrics issued a policy statement supporting CDRTs (American Academy of Pediatrics, 2010). They cite a number of reasons for their support, including legislation which has resulted from CDRT activities, the collection and use of data to emphasize key issues concerning children's health and safety, and increased collaboration between the medical, public health, and law enforcement professions. The Academy also notes the important opportunities to use data to develop a system of surveillance concerning risk factors for and the rate of children's deaths. The Centers for Disease Control and Prevention and others (Leeb, Paulozzi, Melanson, Simon, & Arias, 2008; Schnitzer, Gulino, & Ying-Ying, 2013) have discussed the importance of using data from CDRTs for surveillance of child maltreatment, in general.

Members of the child welfare and social work professions have also heralded the virtues of CDRTs (Riley, 1989), which have been credited with improving the child protection service system, assisting in the development of prevention programs, and influencing social and health policy to help reduce preventable child fatalities (Hochstadt, 2006), even though there is insufficient evidence to support these statements. The professional association, the Child Welfare League of America, recommends conducting (internal) reviews of children's deaths as they provide opportunities for improvements in the child welfare system (Child Welfare League of America, 2007). As with health professionals, social workers have emphasized the unique opportunity to identify risk factors and patterns which may contribute to a child's fatality; additionally some have outlined the unique role for social workers in the CDRT process, which could include conducting interviews of family members and being able to review case records for evidence of child maltreatment or intimate partner violence in the family (Pollack, 2009).

5.6 Outcomes of Child Death Review Teams: Controversy and Success

5.6.1 Common Criticisms

The most consistent criticism of CDRTs in the United States is that they lack uniform policies, reports lack consistency between states (Webster et al., 2003), recommendations are written that do not provide guidance for action (Wirtz et al., 2011), when data collection takes place it varies between states and sometimes even counties, and definitions of what constitutes a fatal child maltreatment varies between counties, regions, and states (Putnam-Hornstein, Wood, Fluke, Yoshioka-Maxwell, & Berger, 2013; Shanley et al., 2010). These are criticisms that are often leveled at the U.S. child welfare system, in general. In truth, many of the critiques about CDRTs themselves are being addressed (Johnston, Bennett, Pilkey, Wirtz, & Quan, 2011). The National Center for the Review and Prevention of Child Deaths provides clear guidance on how to establish a team, develop policy about selecting and conducting reviews, and has implemented the National Child Death Review Case Reporting System which collects state-level CDRT data (Covington, 2011); as of 2011, 35 states were contributing to this system (Covington & Johnston, 2011). This dataset is not, however, a "public use" dataset and is not housed in an archive, such as the National Data Archive on Child Abuse and Neglect. Instead, it is maintained and operated by the National Center for the Review and Prevention of Child Deaths. Thus, it limits opportunities for researchers in the field.

Even with guidance from the National Child Death Review Case Reporting System, it is possible that at the local level CDRTs still experience challenges, such as a lack of resources in time and funding, suspicion that review activities will target individuals, and being resistant to change (Kellermann et al., 1999). As part of writing this chapter, I reached out to the leaders of CDRTs and invited them to speak to me about activities "of note" in their state that might be related to preventing CMFs.[2] One leader told me that his/her state's CDRT was prevented from reviewing any case which had progressed through the criminal justice system, which presumably would be the more serious cases warranting review. A team leader in another state told me that his/her state's child welfare agency refuses to participate in the CDRT activities because they view the work of the CDRT as primary prevention and child welfare agencies are only permitted to engage in activities related to secondary and tertiary prevention (see Chapter 1).

---

[2] Only three CDRT leaders responded and I spoke to all of them. I have kept their identities and the identities of their states confidential.

5.6.2 Lacking Evidence

There has been little research concerning the outcomes and efficacy of CDRTs. At the request of the state's legislative assembly, Kellermann and colleagues conducted an assessment on the efficacy of the then newly established CDRT in the state of Georgia (Kellermann et al., 1999). They reviewed the first 6 years of operation as a way to assess the implementation of CDRTs and to determine if the rate of CMFs had decreased during this time. The authors reported that CDRTs faced significant barriers in implementation of CDR activities throughout the state and that the rate of child deaths had not been affected by the activities of review teams. Six years is likely not enough time to have made an impact on the multiple systems which work to support and protect children and their families, but it might have been enough time to implement CDR activities around the state more completely.

In the United Kingdom and some other countries, there are multiple methods for examining CMFs. Most similar to CDRTs are Child Death Overview Panels (CDOPs), which have a standing body of multidisciplinary professionals who review the deaths of children ("Children Act," 2004; Garstang & Sidebotham, 2008); the United Kingdom also uses the system of instituting public inquiries in which an ad hoc committee examines a mass death or egregious fatality, such as a case of fatal maltreatment where the victim was known to child protective services (Reder, Duncan, & Gray, 1993; Vincent, 2010). CDOPs exist because of a national mandate in England and were implemented in the first decade of the twenty-first century (Sidebotham et al., 2011). The early reviews have been encouraging (Sidebotham et al., 2011), but the recommendations and outcomes of CDOPs have not yet made their way to policy change or measurable outcomes (Allen, Lenton, Fraser, & Sidebotham, 2014; Mazzola et al., 2013).

Public inquiries have been a routine way to "get to the bottom" of CMFs in New Zealand, Australia, and the Netherlands, especially in cases when children and their families were known to protective services (Reder & Duncan, 2004). In this instance, the committee members conduct a thorough investigation about the events leading up to and the circumstances of the child's death. The outcome is a public report in which blame can be, and usually is, ascribed to specific individuals and particular agencies or professional groups (Kuijvenhoven & Kortleven, 2010; Stanley & Manthorpe, 2004; Vincent, 2010), which is distinct from the de-identified reports which emerge from CDRTs/CDOPs. In addition to ascribing blame, the reports which emerge from public inquiries include a series of recommendations for changes in policy and practice that might lead to fewer CMFs (Reder et al., 1993). This latter approach is consistent with CDRTs/CDOPs. Public inquiries have been the subject of criticism, however; some have questioned if public inquiries will ever change the circumstances leading to CMFs (Göpfert, 2009). Other scholars have suggested that taking the lessons learned from the death of one child and generalizing them to the entire child welfare system is inappropriate; problems which may have contributed to a child's death may or may not be relevant to other cases or practice approaches within the child welfare system (Connolly & Doolan, 2007;

Reder & Duncan, 1998). In the United States, there are often "in-house" reviews within child protection agencies when a child dies who is known to protective services. This, too, usually results in recommendations for change (see Washington State Children's Administration, 2008), although the reports do not point fingers at specific individuals and generally draw less media attention than in other countries.

Child welfare scholars have accused some nations of becoming crisis reactive, which results in spending resources on the investigations of deceased children which might be better spent on the primary prevention of child maltreatment (Munro, 2005). The former Commissioner for Children in New Zealand, who is also a pediatrician, has suggested that reviews into children's deaths reduce morale in child protection agencies and can drive agencies into using ineffective, defensive strategies that do not necessarily increase children's well-being (Hassall, 2006). Scholars in the Netherlands conclude that the recommendations which emerge from public inquiries solely focus on bureaucratic and procedural work activities, and will likely never prevent CMFs until there is also a focus on the clinical training, skills, and knowledge of frontline child welfare workers (Kuijvenhoven & Kortleven, 2010; Munro, 2005).

A Scottish government agency undertook a study that examined the review processes for investigating children's deaths—including CDRTs, CDOPs, public inquiries, and other types of review processes—in 14 different countries. According to the rubric that the authors used, the United States performed extremely well, meeting all but one of the identified strengths of reviewing the deaths of children. The authors' ultimate conclusion, however, was that even the best of reviews make a limited contribution toward reforming child protective systems and there is insufficient evidence to say that children will be less likely to die from abuse or neglect. They also argue that recommendations often result in knee-jerk reactions to issues that were relevant to cases ending in death, but might not be relevant to the majority of cases. They state that these reactions tend to be expensive and reinforce an adversarial approach to child welfare work (Axford & Bullock, 2005). On the other hand, a similar international analysis was undertaken, which also largely focused on Scotland. The author of this study argued that important reforms in child protection laws emerged from public inquiries, including the balance between protecting children and parents' rights and the conditions under which a child can be removed from a home, as well as important practice changes, such as child abuse and neglect public awareness campaigns, and the establishment of a 24-hour single national helpline number for reporting maltreatment (Vincent, 2010).

CDRT activities and public inquiries are distinct types of reviews or forms of inquiry into the same type of problem—children dying from maltreatment. Their processes for understanding what led to a CMF are distinct one from another, but their products are similar—recommendations to change a system, a profession, a practice standard, or a policy which may have seemingly contributed to a child's death or limited professionals to take protective action. The public inquiry has been the target of harsh criticism, and it is important to note that countries that use this system of inquiry have more recently moved toward CDRTs/CDOPs, which indicates an interest in doing something beyond a single case review when a child dies from maltreatment. The United States, however, has been included in the criticisms about reactive policy-making approaches to tragedies and a growing dissatisfaction with methods that are seemingly ineffective to promote children's well-being (Mansell, Ota, Erasmus, & Marks, 2011; Munro, 1999, 2005; Parton, 2002).

5.6.3 Bright Spots

There is reason to believe that positive changes may result from reviews; team leaders note the development of prevention programs addressing shaken baby syndrome and infant abandonment, and public education around issues such as water safety (Durfee et al., 2002). A study of CDRT leaders from 41 states showed that CDRT activities resulted in important changes. Team leaders were asked whether CDRT recommendations resulted in action on the state level and to what degree recommendations made an impact on the child protective service system. They found that 91% of states reported acting on the recommendations (68% = some action; 23% = much action) and that 89% reported that the recommendations had an impact on the state's child protection system (72% = some impact; 17% = much impact) (Peddle, Wang, Diaz, & Reid, 2002).

In addition to the Georgia study, the only other study to examine the efficacy of CDRTs was conducted by Palusci and colleagues in Michigan (Palusci, Yager, & Covington, 2010). Their goal was to assess whether CDRT activities resulted in fewer CMFs. Like the study in Georgia (Kellermann et al., 1999), they also used a 6-year time period, 1999–2001 compared with 2002–2004. The authors examined problem areas in child welfare practice that were associated with CMFs from 1999 to 2001, as identified by the state's CDRT. They examined the corrective action that was taken by the state's child welfare system and then determined the rate of CMFs that could still be attributed to those problem areas in 2002–2004. The authors assessed 23 child welfare practice problem areas related to children's deaths, along with a corrective action that was taken for each problem, and found a decline in CMFs in four areas. Those four problem areas where there was a decline in deaths are listed here, followed by the corrective action in parentheses: screening out complaints (implemented new CPS peer review program), time lapse between assignment and contact with families (implemented new CPS peer review program), inaccurate risk assessment completion (implemented statewide CPS training on assessment tools), and record inaccessibility limiting the ability of the child welfare worker to assess the totality of the case (implemented data system upgrades). The authors cautioned against drawing a causal relationship since there were noticeable changes in only four of the 23 problem areas. That said, they did note an overall rate of decline in deaths and a 35% decrease in the number of findings associated with CMFs over this 6-year period. This is a promising way to examine the potential impact of CDRTs on the rate of CMFs.

Additionally, the data collected from CDRTs through the National Child Death Review Case Reporting System are now being aggregated, analyzed, and published in peer-reviewed sources (Palusci & Covington, 2014), even if definitions of CMFs between states continue to differ (Putnam-Hornstein et al., 2013). This data does not provide comparative information, making it impossible to determine how children who die are different from children who live, but it is the first, largest, multi-state and most comprehensive dataset that the United States has on CMF victims and their families (Covington & Johnston, 2011), offering more detailed information about CMFs victims than the National Child Abuse and Neglect Data Set (Schnitzer et al., 2008, 2013).

5.7 The Bottom Line

5.7.1 *What We Know*

The field of CDR has made tremendous strides since it began in the late 1970s in Los Angeles County, California. The following are certainties in this policy and programmatic response to children's deaths:

- Compared to just two decades ago, CDRTs have a strong presence in the United States. Every state in the nation has a CDRT (even if some are fledging and cease to operate from time to time).
- CDRTs are relatively well-supported by legislation, funding, and have been embraced by professional associations. Teams have become institutionalized in many states and settings and are increasingly being used across the globe.
- The composition of state teams is not always consistent with the mission of CDRTs. The primary focus of CDRTs is the prevention of future fatalities, yet the professions which might be most able to have an impact in this area are not always mandated to be at the table: maternal-child health professionals, home visiting professionals, parenting/family life educators, and social workers who work in tandem with child welfare services providing family support services. Researchers are also not members of the team. Instead, these responsibilities tend to be handled by the staff members who coordinate the CDRTs administrative responsibilities or contracted out to individuals outside the team.
- The National Center for the Review and Prevention of Child Deaths has implemented the National Child Death Review Case Reporting System, which is a system for collecting uniform data from CDRTs. At least 35 states provide data. This is the most comprehensive dataset on deceased children in the United States.

5.7.2 *What Remains Unknown*

Despite the tremendous progress made on CDRTs, there continue to be obstacles and a lack of knowledge concerning the effectiveness of CDRTs. One of the most common concerns is the lack of a uniform definition across states regarding what

5.7 The Bottom Line

constitutes a case of fatal maltreatment (Putnam-Hornstein et al., 2013), which makes comparing rates of CMFs between states problematic. This criticism cannot be leveled at CDRTs themselves; definitions of abuse and neglect vary between states and a maltreatment fatality is just an extension of those definitions. CDRTs review whatever cases come before them, regardless of what definitions a state uses. Instead, it would be wise for national leaders to use the expertise of CDRT members to establish national standards for definitions that states could adopt, making it more possible to compare death rates between states and to survey CMFs overtime (Schnitzer et al., 2013).

CDRTs face some barriers at the state and local level. I previously provided some examples based on the conversations that I had with CDRT leadership, which reflect resistance to change, distrust in the CDRT process and goals, and misunderstandings about the focus of CDRTs. Scholars in this area have noted a lack of uniformity in the implementation of CDRT standards at the state and local levels as well (Shanley et al., 2010). Child welfare agencies differ drastically between states and regions, so it is understandable that multiple professions within each state might collectively operate differently between states as well. It is possible that federal legislation might help to streamline and provide increased funding in order to support more uniform implementation of standards for CDRTs. Federal legislation has been proposed, but has not yet passed (Covington & Johnston, 2011).

The most fundamental problems facing CDRTs is the lack of evidence concerning their ability to change policy and practice and to effectively reduce child deaths. One step toward this would be to have CDRTs more consistently issue reports on their activities. My calculations show that only 60.6 % of states issued reports on the activities and recommendations of their CDRT. Even for states that do include this information, details are limited in and not easily tied to actual changes in policy or practice to make children safer. Examples include: "Contribute funding to 'Cribs for Kids' campaign" (Nevada), "Following up on recommendation…to put together social marketing campaign to address safe sleep and car seat safety issues" (Michigan), "Creation of Foster Care Medical Community" (Delaware), and "Made improvements to vision/mission statements and completed a policy and procedure book" (Wyoming). CDRTs could report their achievements, notable activities, changes in child welfare/investigative practice and agency policy, new legislation passed, and other successful activities that they have contributed to—or might contribute to—reducing children's deaths. The National Center for the Review and Prevention of Child Deaths does not currently direct teams to include information about notable activities and achievements as part of their guidelines for writing reports (National Center for the Review and Prevention of Child Deaths, n.d.-a); this might be an important change to make. It would help promote transparency and allow decision-makers and funders to understand the potential benefits of CDR in their state/regions. At the time that this chapter is being written, the National Center for the Review and Prevention of Child Deaths does not currently have a comprehensive listing or report of CDRT successes.

A more significant step would be to track and document the recommendations that are made in CDRT reports. As it stands, recommendations are made and there is no evidence that they are acted on or monitored. In fact, one report that I read issued the same recommendations annually, regardless of the deaths or problems that were reviewed each year. If states were to follow the recommendations issued, they would report on the progress made in realizing the recommendations issued in prior reports. In order to accomplish such a task, a CDRT would need to follow the work of Wirtz and colleagues (Wirtz et al., 2011) and include the individuals or parties responsible for monitoring the outcomes of recommendations issued by CDRTs (see Table 5.3 for a refresher on this topic).

The most significant leap would be to determine if there is a connection between CDRT activities and recommendations, and rates of CMFs in the same state. For example, can the implementation of new training, practice standards, child welfare agency policy, or state policy be linked to a change—presumably a decline—in the rate of CMFs?[3] The most effective way to determine a link between an intervention and an outcome is to take an approach that is similar to what Palusci and colleagues undertook (Palusci et al., 2010). As previously discussed, they compared actions taken to correct identified problem areas in child welfare practice and then compared whether there was a change over time in CMFs attributed to those problems. In this way, it is possible to identify whether changes in a particular area of social work, medicine, or the criminal justice system contribute to a specific change in the rate of CMFs. It would, presumably, be a less overwhelming task for CDRTs than trying to determine which of their varied activities might, or might not, have an effect on the rate of CMFs.

In conclusion, CDRTs offer significant promise in their ability to bring change in the prevention, intervention, and handling of CMFs. Despite challenges to the culture of some professional groups or individuals, there is widespread support for CDRTs and a belief that their methods work to prevent CMFs (Covington & Johnston, 2011). In fact, their methods may prevent CMFs, but the evidence to show that is largely lacking. The rate of CMFs has risen over the period of time that CDRTs have been implemented (see Chapter 2). That rise may, in fact, be the result of CDRTs' work to encourage professionals in the field to more accurately identify cases of CMFs, making it appear that the rate of CMFs is increasing, when in truth the field is finally able to more accurately determine the prevalence of the problem. At this point, however, this is primarily speculation and in a theme that is repeated throughout this book, the bottom line is that we don't really know if the time, resources, and expertise that we have invested in CDRTs is paying off without more effectively evaluating our efforts.

---

[3] It can be tempting for CDRTs to only document the number of children who died each year. Reporting the rate is the more appropriate figure because the number of children in a state changes annually, so it is important to know the proportion of children who die each year as opposed to only the numbers. One state made a potential connection between a home visiting program and a decline in the number of CMF victims each year; reporting the rate would have made their argument more convincing to readers and to decision-makers.

References

Allen, L., Lenton, S., Fraser, J., & Sidebotham, P. (2014). Improving the practice of child death overview panels: A paediatric perspective. *Archives of Disease in Childhood, 99*(3), 193–196. doi:10.1136/archdischild-2013-305085.

American Academy of Pediatrics. (2010). Policy statement – Child fatality review. *Pediatrics, 126*(3), 592–596. doi:10.1542/peds.2010-2006.

Axford, N., & Bullock, R. (2005). *Child death and significant case reviews: International approaches.* Dartington Social Research Unit.

Berkowitz, C. D. (2008). Child abuse recognition and reporting: Supports and resources for changing the paradigm. *Pediatrics, 122*(Suppl 1), S10–S12.

Brandon, M., Dodsworth, J., & Rumball, D. (2005). Serious case reviews: Learning to use expertise. *Child Abuse Review, 14*(3), 160–176.

Bunting, L., & Reid, C. (2005). Reviewing child deaths--Learning from the American experience. *Child Abuse Review, 14*(2), 82–96.

Child Welfare League of America, I. (2007). Eye on CWLA: Using the special review as a program improvement tool. *Children's Voice*, September/October.

Children Act, Great Britain, Her Majesty Government Stat. (2004).

Children's Health Alliance of Wisconsin. (2010). *A window into prevention: An initial report on preventing child death & injury in Wisconsin.* Retrieved January 4, 2015, from http://www.childdeathreview.org/Reports/WI_FullRpt2010.pdf

Connolly, M., & Doolan, M. (2007). Responding to the deaths of children known to child protection agencies. *Social Policy Journal of New Zealand, 30*, 1–11.

Covington, T., & Johnston, B. (2011). A misdirected assessment of progress in child death review. *American Journal of Preventive Medicine, 40*(5), e31. doi:10.1016/j.amepre.2011.01.011.

Covington, T. M. (2011). The US National Child Death review case reporting system. *Injury Prevention: Journal of the International Society for Child and Adolescent Injury Prevention, 17*(Suppl 1), i34–i37. doi:10.1136/ip.2010.031203.

Devaney, J., Lazenbatt, A., & Bunting, L. (2011). Inquiring into non-accidental child deaths: Reviewing the review process. *British Journal of Social Work, 41*(2), 242–260. doi:10.1093/bjsw/bcq069.

Douglas, E. M. (2005). Child maltreatment fatalities: What do we know, what have we done and where do we go from here? In K. Kendall-Tackett & S. Gaicomoni (Eds.), *Child victimization* (pp. 4.1–4.18). Kingston, NJ: Civic Research Institute.

Douglas, E. M., & Cunningham, J. M. (2008). Recommendations from child fatality review teams: results of a US nationwide exploratory study concerning maltreatment fatalities and social service delivery. *Child Abuse Review, 17*(5), 331–351. doi:10.1002/car.1044.

Douglas, E. M., & McCarthy, S. C. (2011). Child fatality review teams: A content analysis of social policy. *Child Welfare, 90*(3), 91–110.

Durfee, M., Durfee, D. T., & West, M. P. (2002). Child fatality review: An international movement. *Child Abuse & Neglect, 26*, 619–636.

Durfee, M., Parra, J. M., & Alexander, R. (2009). Child fatality review teams. *Pediatric Clinics of North America, 56*(2), 379–387. doi:10.1016/j.pcl.2009.01.004.

Durfee, M. J., & Durfee, D. T. (1995). Multi-agency child death review teams: Experience in the United States. *Child Abuse Review, 4*, 377–381.

Durfee, M. J., Gellert, G. A., & Durfee, D. T. (1992). Origins and clinical relevance of child death review teams. *JAMA, 267*(23), 3172–3175.

Garstang, J., & Sidebotham, P. (2008). Interagency training: Establishing a course in the management of unexpected childhood death. *Child Abuse Review, 17*(5), 352–361.

Gellert, G. A., Maxwell, R. M., Durfee, M. J., & Wagner, G. A. (1995). Fatalities assessed by the orange county child death review team, 1989 to 1991. *Child Abuse & Neglect, 19*(7), 875–883.

Göpfert, M. (2009). Guest Editorial: A message from Britain: Inquiries into child deaths – Will it ever change? *Advances in Mental Health, 8*(3), 227–230. doi:10.5172/jamh.8.3.227.

Hassall, I. (2006). What is to be done about child homicide in New Zealand?
Hochstadt, N. J. (2006). Child death review teams: A vital component of child protection. *Child Welfare, 85*(4), 653–670.
Johnston, B. D., Bennett, E., Pilkey, D., Wirtz, S. J., & Quan, L. (2011). Collaborative process improvement to enhance injury prevention in child death review. *Injury Prevention, 17*, 71–76.
Kellermann, A. L., Thomas, W., Henry, G., Wald, M., Fajman, N. N., & Carter, J. (1999). *The best intentions: An evaluation of the child fatality review process in Georgia*. Retrieved October 12, 2003, 2003, from http://www.sph.emory.edu/CIC/gafatality.html
Kuijvenhoven, T., & Kortleven, W. J. (2010). Inquiries into fatal child abuse in the Netherlands: A source of improvement? *British Journal of Social Work, 40*(4), 1152–1173. doi:10.1093/bjsw/bcq014.
Leeb, R. T., Paulozzi, L. J., Melanson, C., Simon, T. R., & Arias, I. (2008). *Child maltreatment surveillance: Uniform definitions for public health and recommended data elements*. Atlanta, GA: Centers for Disease Control & Prevention. Retrieved from http://www.cdc.gov/violenceprevention/pdf/cm_surveillance-a.pdf
Luallen, J. J., Rochat, R. W., Smith, S. M., O'Neil, J., Rogers, M. Y., & Bolen, J. C. (1998). Child fatality review in Georgia: A young system demonstrates its potential for identifying preventable childhood deaths. *South Medical Journal, 91*(5), 414–419.
Mansell, J., Ota, R., Erasmus, R., & Marks, K. (2011). Reframing child protection: A response to a constant crisis of confidence in child protection. *Children and Youth Services Review, 33*(11), 2076–2086. doi:10.1016/j.childyouth.2011.04.019.
Mazzola, F., Mohiddin, A., Ward, M., & Holdsworth, G. (2013). How useful are child death reviews: A local area's perspective. *BMC Research Notes, 6*(1), 295–295.
Munro, E. (2005). Improving practice: Child protection as a systems problem. *Children and Youth Services Review, 27*(4), 375–391.
Munro, E. M. (1999). Protecting children in an anxious society. *Health, Risk & Society, 1*(1), 117–127.
National Center for the Review and Prevention of Child Deaths. (2010). *The status of child death review in the United States in 2009*. Updated July 2010.
National Center for the Review and Prevention of Child Deaths. (n.d.-a). *CDR reporting*. Retrieved March 28, 2014, from http://www.childdeathreview.org/reporting.htm
National Center for the Review and Prevention of Child Deaths. (n.d.-b). *State spotlights*. Retrieved March 4, 2014, from http://www.childdeathreview.org/state.htm
Palusci, V. J., & Covington, T. M. (2014). Child maltreatment deaths in the U.S. National Child Death Review Case Reporting System. *Child Abuse & Neglect, 38*(1), 25–36. doi:http://dx.doi.org/10.1016/j.chiabu.2013.08.014.
Palusci, V. J., Yager, S., & Covington, T. M. (2010). Effects of a Citizens Review Panel in preventing child maltreatment fatalities. *Child Abuse & Neglect, 34*(5), 324–331.
Parton, N. (2002). Narrow, restrictive and reactive. *Community Care, 1410*, 24.
Peddle, N., Wang, C.-T., Diaz, J., & Reid, R. (2002). *Current trends in child abuse prevention and fatalities: The 2000 Fifty State Survey* (Working paper no. 808). Retrieved September 1, 2008, from http://www.pcao.org/resources/pdfs/2000_50_survey.pdf
Pennsylvania Bureau of Family Health. (2013). *Pennsylvania child death review annual report*. Retrieved January 4, 2015, from http://www.portal.state.pa.us/portal/server.pt/gateway/PTARGS_0_75878_1403057_0_0_18/PA_CDR_2013_Annual_Report_Final_w_Errata_Edits.pdf
Pollack, D. (2009). Child fatality review teams and the role of social workers: An international perspective. *International Social Work, 52*(2), 247–253.
Putnam-Hornstein, E., Wood, J. N., Fluke, J., Yoshioka-Maxwell, A., & Berger, R. P. (2013). Preventing severe and fatal child maltreatment: Making the case for the expanded use and integration of data. *Child Welfare, 92*(2), 59–75.
Reder, P., & Duncan, S. (1998). A proposed system for reviewing child abuse deaths. *Child Abuse Review, 7*, 280–286.

References

Reder, P., & Duncan, S. (1999). *Lost innocents: A follow-up study of fatal child abuse*. Florence, KY: Taylor & Frances/Routledge.

Reder, P., & Duncan, S. (2004). Making the most of the Victoria Climbié Inquiry Report. *Child Abuse Review, 13*(2), 95–114. doi:10.1002/car.834.

Reder, P., Duncan, S., & Gray, M. (1993). *Beyond blame: Child abuse tragedies revisited*. London, UK: Taylor & Frances/Routledge.

Riley, J. W. (1989). Child fatalities review process. *Protecting Children, 6*(1), 6–8.

Schnitzer, P. G., Covington, T. M., Wirtz, S. J., Verhoek-Oftedahl, W., & Palusci, V. J. (2008). Public health surveillance of fatal child maltreatment: Analysis of 3 state programs. *American Journal of Public Health, 98*(2), 296–303. doi:10.2105/ajph.2006.087783.

Schnitzer, P. G., Gulino, S. P., & Ying-Ying, T. Y. (2013). Advancing public health surveillance to estimate child maltreatment fatalities: Review and recommendations. *Child Welfare, 92*(2), 77–98.

Shanley, J. R., Risch, E. C., & Bonner, B. L. (2010). U.S. child death review programs: Assessing progress toward a standard review process. *American Journal of Preventive Medicine, 39*(6), 522–528. doi:10.1016/j.amepre.2010.08.010.

Sidebotham, P., Fox, J., Horwath, J., & Powell, C. (2011). Developing effective child death review: A study of 'early starter' child death overview panels in England. *Injury Prevention: Journal of the International Society for Child and Adolescent Injury Prevention, 17*(Suppl 1), i55–i63. doi:10.1136/ip.2010.027169.

Stanley, N., & Manthorpe, J. (2004). The inquiry as Janus. In N. Stanley & J. Manthorpe (Eds.), *The age of the inquiry. Learning and blaming in health and social care* (pp. 1–16). London, UK: Routledge.

Texas Child Fatality Review Team. (2011). *Texas child fatality review team report*. Retrieved January 4, 2015, from http://www.childdeathreview.org/reports/TX_CFRAnnualReport2011.pdf

Theiss-Nyland, K., & Rechel, B. (2013). *Death reviews: Maternal, perinatal and child PMNCH knowledge summary* (Vol. 27). Geneva, Switzerland: The Partnership for Maternal, Newborn and Child Health.

U.S. Department of Health & Human Services. (n.d.). *Healthy people 2020: Injury and violence prevention*. Washington, DC. Retrieved from http://www.healthypeople.gov/2020/topicsobjectives2020/objectiveslist.aspx?topicid=24

Utah Department of Health. (2010). *Child injury deaths in Utah, 2005–2007*. Retrieved January 4, 2015, from http://www.health.utah.gov/vipp/pdf/ChildFatality/ChildInjuryDeathsReport.pdf

Vincent, S. (2010). *Preventing child deaths: Learning from review*. Edinburgh, UK: Dunedin Academic Press Ltd.

Ward Platt, M. (2014). Child death review five years on. *Archives of Disease in Childhood, 99*(3), 187–188. doi:10.1136/archdischild-2013-305707.

Washington State Children's Administration. (2008). *Children's administration executive child fatality review: Saranadee Leingang*. Department of Social and Health Services. Retrieved from http://www.dshs.wa.gov/pdf/ca/LeingangECFR.pdf

Webster, R. A., Schnitzer, P. G., Jenny, C., Ewigman, B. G., & Alario, A. J. (2003). Child death review: The state of the nation. *American Journal of Preventive Medicine, 25*(5), 58–64.

Wirtz, S. J., Foster, V., & Lenart, G. A. (2011). Assessing and improving child death review team recommendations. *Injury Prevention, 17*, 64–70.

Chapter 6
State Safe Haven Laws

Sometimes parents abandon or discard infants very early in life and this often leads to death. The reasons for and circumstances under which parents do this are varied, but in most circumstances, this is generally considered a form of physical neglect. The most universal response to this in the United States has been to pass "safe haven" laws—or laws that allow parents to legally relinquish infants in designated areas without any criminal consequences. Undoubtedly, this is one of the most popular responses to fatal child maltreatment discussed in this book. All states in the U.S. have safe haven laws. This chapter will discuss the history, purpose, and use of these laws. I also highlight the central controversies associated with or limitations of safe haven laws here and expand on them in the body of the chapter.

- There is no centralized way to track the use or effectiveness of safe haven laws. For example, it is impossible to know how many infants were abandoned in the United States in a given year, let alone how many infants were relinquished to a safe haven location. Some states track this information, but there is no national registry for tracking abandonment or safe haven relinquishments.
- In order for safe haven laws to work at even the most basic level, expectant parents and the general public need to know about them. There is little evidence that there is widespread knowledge about safe haven laws.
- When public education about safe haven laws is employed, it is primarily marketed to young, teenage mothers, but there is reason to believe that infant abandonment happens among mothers of all child-bearing years.
- Safe haven laws have been criticized as the "least difficult" and least expensive action to take against preventing fatal child maltreatment. State legislators pass laws permitting new parents to relinquish their infants, but this action is not met with legislation to prevent unwanted pregnancies and to prevent parents from being in a position where they feel the need to relinquish their infants.
- Safe haven laws pose unique challenges regarding the parental rights of both parents. For example, if a mother relinquishes a newborn and does not disclose any information about herself or the child's father, the state may move toward adoption without termination of parental rights from the father.

© Springer Science+Business Media Dordrecht 2017
E.M. Douglas, *Child Maltreatment Fatalities in the United States*,
DOI 10.1007/978-94-017-7583-0_6

6.1 The Problem of Abandoned and Discarded Infants

Each year, dozens of infants are abandoned or discarded by their parents or another caregiver. These children are left in dumpsters, trash cans, toilets, bathroom floors, doorsteps, alleys, cemeteries, open fields, the woods, sides of the road, and other inhospitable locations (Pruitt, 2008). In some instances, someone discovers these infants before they die and are rushed to medical services and survive. Other infants are not so lucky and are discovered after their death. Sometimes infants are killed by a caregiver shortly after birth and their bodies are discarded after the killing (Meyer, Oberman, & Rone, 2001; U.S. Department of Health & Human Services, 1998). There are also infants who are discarded each year who are never discovered by anyone; only the parents know of their births and abandonments.

There are several different types of infant abandonment. *Boarder babies* or *abandoned babies* are infants who are left in hospitals after birth, often by drug-addicted mothers because a child welfare agency has determined that the infant cannot go into his/her parents' care. These babies ultimately go into the care of the state. *Discarded babies* are infants who are left in alleys, trashcans, dumpsters, church steps, or another public place without adequate supervision. These infants are sometimes discovered while still alive; other times they are discarded and die; finally, others are killed prior to being discarded (U.S. Department of Health & Human Services, 1998). In this chapter, I mostly address infants who are discarded and die or infants who are killed by their parents and then discarded. Despite the technical definitions used by the U.S. Department of Health & Human Services, I use the terms "abandon" and "discard" interchangeably to discuss infants (alive or deceased) who are left in public places. This choice of words is consistent with language in state statute, the media, and public education campaigns about safe haven laws.

Text Box 6.1
Dinwiddie County, Virginia: "Small, who was originally charged with first-degree murder in the death of her newborn, was found guilty on the lesser charge of involuntary manslaughter. The 22-year-old walked out of the Dinwiddie Circuit Courthouse a free woman after entering her guilty plea. She was sentenced to three years, with three years suspended…Small was charged in October 2013 after she gave birth to the child while sitting on a toilet inside her Namozine Road home. In court Wednesday it was revealed the autopsy showed drowning was the cause of death for the newborn. However, defense attorney Joe Morrissey told CBS 6 reporter Jerrita Patterson that the baby girl's death was an 'accidental killing.' Morrissey said Small did not know she was pregnant, adding his client was planning to take a pregnancy test when she unexpectedly gave birth to a nearly full-term baby" (Patterson, 2014).

6.1 The Problem of Abandoned and Discarded Infants

Infants are generally abandoned by parents who are in duress or parents who lack the ability to care for an infant. Some teenage girls or women describe not realizing that they are pregnant; they report having felt sick, having gone to the bathroom, and then discover a baby in the toilet, as described in Text Box 6.1. These women describe being shocked, afraid, and even disgusted by what they see and flee the scene. Other expectant mothers describe keeping their pregnancy a secret from everyone in their lives. These women are often socially isolated, lack social support, or fear anger from family members or the father of the baby. They usually go through labor alone and discard the baby without assistance from others. Still other women who have openly acknowledged their pregnancy describe situations where they, too, experience labor without the assistance of medical providers and discard their infants with or without help or knowledge of others. They tell family members that they lost the baby or that the baby was a still birth (McKee, 2006; Meyer et al., 2001). There have also recently been stories in the media about mothers abandoning infants that are older, including 5 ("Baby left overnight in woods; mother held," 2014) and 8 month-old infants (Rafferty, 2013). Finally, sometimes when an infant is discarded, the parents kill the child before disposing or discarding of the body, as described in Text Box 6.2. This can happen in conjunction with any of the circumstances already described thus far (Herman-Giddens, Smith, Mittal, Carlson, & Butts, 2003).

Text Box 6.2
San Antonio, Texas: "In the days before the short life of 'Baby Boy Mendoza' ended with the 3-day-old strangled and discarded in the trash, Nidia Yolibeth Alvarado indicated she didn't want another child...[S]he remained in jail charged with capital murder. Two relatives who dropped her off at the hospital told police they didn't know she was pregnant until she asked for a ride there. A day after relatives picked her up, the infant's body would be found on a conveyor belt at an East Side recycling center—inside a duffel bag Alvarado had received from the hospital... Alvarado, 25, was arrested at her North Side apartment late Tuesday. Her bail was set at $2 million. 'The defendant said she ... killed the baby by wrapping a ligature around the baby's neck,' a detective said in an arrest warrant affidavit. Alvarado 'stated she saw the baby was crying and she then saw it die'." (Mondo, 2014)

Determining the magnitude of infant abandonment in the United States is another piece of this puzzle. The United States does not have a method for counting abandoned or discarded infants (Oberman, 2008). In fact, most states lack a system for tracking the number of infants who are abandoned each year. There are only a handful of studies of abandoned and discarded infants. There were two studies commissioned by the U.S. Department of Health and Human Services to assess the scope of abandoned and discarded infants (U.S. Department of Health & Human Services,

1994, 1998). Accounts of deceased infants were taken from news stories using the LexisNexis database and compiled for examination. Of the infants who were found discarded, 65 in 1992 and 105 in 1997; not all were deceased: eight in 1992 and 33 in 1997. With such small numbers and limited methodology, it is impossible to say whether there was an actual increase in number of discarded and deceased children during this timeframe, or whether the increase in numbers is a result of increased reporting on the issue or a change in the numbers of newspapers in the LexisNexis database.

The most carefully constructed study was conducted in North Carolina using the records from the medical examiner's office of 34 infants who were abandoned and deceased when they were discovered between 1985 and 2000 (Herman-Giddens et al., 2003). A second study was conducted in Texas using newspaper accounts of 93 infants who were abandoned in that state between 1996 and 2006; 17 of these infants were found after they were deceased (Pruitt, 2008). These studies show that discarded infants die from a variety of causes, including asphyxiation/strangulation, drowning, hypothermia/exposure, prematurity/lack of care, stabbing, blunt trauma, and heart defect (Herman-Giddens et al., 2003). Both North Carolina and Texas have racially and ethnically diverse populations and that was reflected among the infants that were abandoned; further, these two studies showed that males may be more likely to be abandoned than females (Herman-Giddens et al., 2003; Pruitt, 2008).

6.2 History of Infant Abandonment and Safe Haven Laws

Relinquishing a child out of desperation, or any other reason, has a lengthy history both inside and outside of the United States. For hundreds of years, infants have been abandoned on church steps, hospitals, sidewalks, the woods, and other public places. Many times infants were relinquished in places where someone would find them and provide them with care. In fact, in the middle ages, infant abandonment was such an issue that some countries established "foundling wheels," which were small barrels on a wheel that were placed in an opening of a building, such as in nunneries, hospitals, orphanages and the like. A parent standing outside the building would place an infant in the barrel, turn the wheel, and the occupants on the other side of the wall would receive the infant. These depositories were also sometimes called "baby hatches" or "baby drops" (Kertzer, 1991; Tilly, Fuchs, Kertzer, & Ransel, 1992). These were prominent throughout European countries, Russia and other nations. There were even foundling hospitals devoted exclusively for caring for abandoned infants. According to historical research, at one point in the middle of the 1800s, two institutions in St. Petersburg and Moscow, Russia were taking in 26,000 infants annually (Tilly et al., 1992). The rise in social welfare programs at the end of the nineteenth and into the middle of the twentieth centuries eventually lead countries to turn away from anonymous infant abandonment.

The crack cocaine epidemic, HIV-affected babies, and a rise in discarded infants brought this issue back to the table in the 1980s (Curran & Pletrzak, 2001). The first legislative action taken to address abandoned infants in the United States was the federal Abandoned Infants Assistance Act, which passed in the U.S. Congress in 1988. This law primarily targets the medical care and family needs of infants abandoned in hospitals and there is also a heavy emphasis on HIV or drug-affected infants ("Abandoned Infants Assistance Act," 1988). The law provided funding for demonstration programs that has provided resources, training, and technical support to those in the field (Curran & Pletrzak, 2001). One of the resource centers which resulted from this legislation, the National Abandoned Infants Assistance Resource Center (2005), does devote some attention to discarded infants, but the law itself has not focused on preventing death or infant discarding and therefore, is not a primary focus in this chapter.

The rise in popularity of laws in the United States that would allow parents to relinquish an infant started in Mobile, Alabama. In the wake of dealing with numerous cases of infant abandonment, a local news reporter, Jodi Brooks, and the then-district attorney, John Tyson, Jr., started a "Secret Place for Newborns" in 1998 (Carter, 2013; *Recognizing Mobile County district attorney John Tyson and his work in creating the Alabama Secret Safe Place program*, 2008). This program allowed mothers to legally relinquish an infant up to 3 days old to medical staff at a hospital. Meanwhile, on Long Island, New York, immediately outside of New York City, law enforcement paramedic, Timothy Jaccard was on the scene when multiple abandoned and deceased infants were discovered. This prompted him to dedicate his life, full-time, to recognizing discarded infants who perished, by giving them funerals and appropriate burials. He also set on a mission to get a "safe haven law" passed in his home state of New York. Such a law would allow a parent to legally relinquish an infant to a designated professional, without fear of criminal prosecution. When he was unable to make progress in New York, he heard that Texas was having a similar problem with abandoned infants. He flew to Texas and met with then-governor George W. Bush, who threw his full support behind safe haven legislation, which was passed in 1999 (Jaccard, 2014; Tebo, 2001). The Texas safe haven law was termed "Baby Moses"—referencing the Biblical figure who, as an infant, was found floating in a basket on a river without any supervision. The Texas law allowed parents of infants up to 60 days old to relinquish their children at a hospital or with emergency medical staff or at a welfare office without suffering criminal prosecution (Tebo, 2001). With the continued guidance, dedication, and advocacy of Timothy Jaccard, within 10 years, all of the states in the United States, including our nation's capital, the District of Columbia, had adopted a similar version of safe haven legislation ("D.C. Council OKs newborn safe haven," 2009; Domash, Gallucci, & Twarowski, 2010; T. Jaccard, Personal communication, November 15, 2014).

6.2.1 The Specifics of Safe Haven Laws

Safe haven laws permit parents to safely relinquish an infant at a designated place where the infant will be protected and then turned over to child protective services (Appell, 2002a). To safely relinquish an infant means to leave an infant at a location

Table 6.1 Locations Where Infants Can Be Relinquished, by Descending Order of Frequency[a]

Locations Where Infant Can Be Relinquished	Number of States Indicating
Hospital	49
Emergency medical staff	32
Fire department	28
Police	25
Medical clinic	17
Birthing center	13
Welfare agency	6
Church	4
Health department	4
Adoption clinic	3
Responsible adult	2

[a]Not mutually exclusive categories

that is designated by state statute, in the care of a professional or other designated individual. The infant must be free from signs of abuse or neglect at the time of relinquishment. This action prompts the termination of parental rights to the child, thus, the state works to prepare the child for adoption. Safe haven laws protect parents from criminal prosecution of child abandonment. The laws have been viewed as a win-win: infants are not abandoned in circumstances that might lead to the child's death, parents avoid criminal prosecution, and a family adopts an infant that moves through the legal system relatively quickly. Their efficacy has been questioned, however (Hammond, Miller, & Griffin, 2010).

The National Safe Haven Alliance (n.d.) and the Child Welfare Information Gateway (2010) both provide information on safe haven laws, including specific details about each state statute. In 2013–2014, a colleague and I examined the scope and breadth of safe haven laws in all 50 states, plus the District of Columbia, to determine the locations where infants can be relinquished, the ages at which infants can be relinquished, and who may relish children (Douglas & Mohn, 2014). We found that state statute allows children to be relinquished in a variety of locations: adoption clinics, birthing centers, churches, emergency medical staff, fire departments, health departments, hospitals/emergency rooms, medical clinics, police departments, a responsible adult, and welfare agencies. State statutes most often specify that infants can be relinquished to staff at hospitals/emergency rooms, emergency medical staff, fire departments or police departments. Table 6.1 displays the frequency with which each location is mentioned in state law. On average, states designate three to four locations where an infant can be safely relinquished. Figure 6.1 provides an example of a placard that would be posted at a safe haven location.

Infants can be relinquished when they are between the ages of immediate newborn, up to 1 year of life, depending on the state in which the infant is relinquished. Table 6.2 shows the ages during which infants can be relinquished according to state statute. Most states stipulate that an infant can be relinquished between "up to 72

Figure 6.1 Example of Baby Safe Haven Placard, provided by Save Abandoned Babies Foundation in Illinois

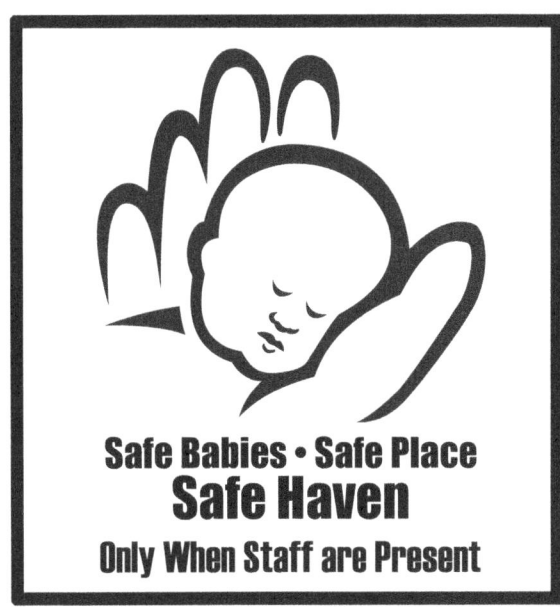

Table 6.2 Ages During Which Infants Can Be Relinquished, by Age of the Child

Age Categories	Number of States Indicating
Up to 3 days	14
Up to 1 week	7
Up to 2 weeks	4
Up to 3 weeks	1
Up to 1 month	19
Up to 1.5 months	1
Up to 2 months	2
Up to 3 months	1
Up to 1 year	2

hours" old and 1 month old. States that allow children to be relinquished at older ages include Texas and South Dakota at 60 days old, New Mexico at 90 days old, and North Dakota and Missouri at 1 year of age.

Safe haven laws also specify who can legally relinquish an infant to a designated location. State statute most often references "parents" as those designated to relinquish a child, but some states also specify that an "agent of the parent" can relinquish a child. Other states only specify that "a person" can relinquish a child and do not place any limits on who that person must be. Six states specify that only the mother or an individual who has the mother's permission can relinquish a child; finally, two states indicate that the only person who can relinquish a child, is a person who has legal custody of the child. Table 6.3 shows the frequency with which

Table 6.3 Who Has Legal Authority to Relinquish Child, by Descending Order of Frequency[a]

Who Has Legal Authority to Relinquish Child?	Number of States Indicating
Parent	46
Agent of parent	12
A person	10
Mother only/Has mother's approval	6
Person with custody of child	2

[a]Are not mutually exclusive categories

these individuals are specified in state statute. Below are examples of language from state legislation.

> *Example of Parent or Agent of Parent:* "If a *parent* or *agent of a parent* voluntarily delivers the parent's newborn infant to a safe haven provider, the safe haven provider shall take custody of the newborn infant." (Arizona Revised Statutes, §13-3623.01)
>
> *Example of Person:* "A *person* may leave a newborn child with the personnel of a hospital, fire station, or police station or emergency services personnel without being subject to prosecution for abandonment of a child…" (Hawaii Revised Statutes, §587-D)
>
> *Example of Mother Only/Mother's Approval:* "[Infant] is voluntarily left by a person who purported to be the *child's mother* and who did not express an intension of returning for the infant…" (Tennessee Code Annotated, §36-1-142)
>
> *Example of Custody of Child:* "A parent or other person having *lawful custody* of an infant which is 45 days old or younger and which has not suffered bodily harm may surrender physical custody of the infant…" (Kansas Statutes Annotated, §38-2282)

One of the key components of safe haven legislation is that parents can relinquish a child anonymously with no questions asked. There is significant variation between states in how this provision is handled, but it is largely true—an infant can be surrendered to a safe haven location and the relinquisher can walk away. Some states do encourage staff at safe haven locations to urge relinquishing parents to provide information about the child's medical history or to learn if there are other children at home who might be at-risk in some way, but most states do not. Here is one example:

> *Example of Responsibility of Safe Haven Provider:* On taking possession of a child, a law enforcement agency, hospital, or emergency medical service organization shall do…the following…If possible, make forms available to the parents who delivered the child to gather medical information concerning the child and the child's parents. (Ohio, Revised Statute, §2151.3517)

The primary hook of safe haven laws that is supposed to be most appealing to parents who have an infant that they want to relinquish, is that they will not be prosecuted for surrendering their child. Specifically, they will not be criminally or civilly prosecuted for child abandonment, child neglect, child abuse, endangering the welfare of a child, or other similar charges. States have handled this in a variety

6.2 History of Infant Abandonment and Safe Haven Laws

of ways. Some states provide an "affirmative defense"[1] against the types of criminal charges that might follow charges of infant abandonment. In these states a parent might still be charged with criminal abandonment, neglect, or abuse, but as long as the parent followed the procedures outlined in safe haven legislation, that parent would have an affirmative defense to such charges and be cleared of any wrongdoing. Other states provide a shield against prosecution of criminal charges against a parent safely relinquishing a child to a safe haven location. Finally, in a small number of states, safe haven relinquishments are exempt from the definitions of criminal neglect, abuse, or abandonment (Appell, 2002a). Here are some examples of language declaring protection from criminal prosecution in state statute.

Example of Affirmative Defense: Relinquishment to a safe haven is an affirmative defense to prosecution for nonsupport, abandonment, or endangering the welfare of a child. (Alabama Code, §26-25-3)

Example of Shield Against Prosecution: A person who leaves an infant at a hospital or other facility, or directs another person to do so, shall be immune from prosecution only for the act of abandonment of the infant… (Rhode Island General Laws, §22-13.1-.4)

Example of Exemptions in Definition: It is not a crime for a parent to deliver a child to an emergency medical services provider or a licensed child-placing agency if the child has not been harmed prior to being left with the emergency medical services provider or a licensed child-placing agency. (South Dakota, Annotated Laws §§ 25-5A-28)

In our analyses of the different components of safe haven laws, we found that there is tremendous variation between states. That said, we found no regional variations with regard to the limit on a child's age, who can relinquish a child, and where a child can be relinquished. I have found the same phenomenon to be true in my research on state-level social policies to assist or support families or divorce or disruption; there were no regional patterns to explain or understand the laws that were pass (Douglas, 2006). In fact, I was once presenting said research at a conference filled with political scientists and one person in the audience openly said, "I've never even seen state policy maps that look anything like these laws." The same appears to be true with safe haven laws.

The only state characteristics that we found to be related to safe haven laws were the rate at which children die from abuse or neglect and state unemployment. When maltreatment fatality rates were higher, as well as unemployment rates, states were less likely to pass legislation allowing someone other than a parent to relinquish an infant. Readers should keep in mind, however, that only a total of five states allow someone other than the child's parent to relinquish an infant.

---

[1] According to Cornell University's online legal dictionary, Wex, an "affirmative defense" is "a defense in which the defendant introduces evidence, which, if found to be credible, will negate criminal or civil liability, even if it is proven that the defendant committed the alleged acts." In addition to safe haven laws, other examples of affirmative defenses include self-defense or insanity.

6.3 What if Safe Haven Laws Did Not Exist?

Safe haven laws are relatively new in the United States, but it is worth exploring the alternatives to safe haven laws. What if they did not exist? What other options could parents pursue once they are near the delivery date for a pregnancy or once an unwanted infant has been delivered? If parents were at risk of harming their children, they could call child protective services and ask for their child to be removed. In such an instance, the parents might be substantiated for threat of harm for abuse or neglect, but could not be prosecuted for criminal abandonment, since no abandonment would have taken place. Child welfare professionals would work with those parents to see if they were in need of more supports and what other family might exist who could care for the child. If a parent was not at risk of harming his or her child, but simply wanted to relinquish the child from his/her care, the child protective agency would likely refer that parent to an adoption agency (Pollock & Hittle, 2003). Other options would be for parents to take a more traditional route of identifying and working with an adoption agency to find a permanent home and legal parents for the child (Appell, 2002b). As outlined by the Child Welfare League of America, parents who have unwanted pregnancies and infants, can and do receive support from a variety of different sources, including schools, churches, healthcare providers, and as already noted, public child welfare agencies and private adoption agencies (Pollock & Hittle, 2003). The League argues that parents who discard an infant have not received adequate support from these existing community resources.

6.4 Common Concerns About Safe Haven Laws

6.4.1 *Efficacy of Safe Haven Laws*

There is very little research that has examined the efficacy of safe haven laws (Deoudes, 2003). In order for the laws to be effective, knowledge of their existence is required. Babies *are* being relinquished through safe haven locations (Ontiveros, 2014), so clearly there is some public knowledge about the existence of safe haven laws. Beyond this, there is almost no measure of knowledge among expecting parents, safe haven receivers, or the general public. One study assessed knowledge of safe haven laws among emergency medicine residents in New York City (Ryan, Caputo, & Berrett, 2014). Knowledge about the existence of safe haven laws was below 20% among first year residents, but was about 50% among fourth year residents, indicating a likely increase in awareness of laws over the course of their training. Knowledge concerning the specifics of the law, such as locations for relinquishment and age limits, hovered around 20% for all residents, regardless of the year of their training. This one study reinforces anecdotal evidence that there is a general lack of awareness about safe haven laws and the options that they provide to new parents (Hensley, 2013; Ranney, 2010). According to the Chicago-based Save Abandoned Babies Foundation in Chicago, Illinois, their state now requires high schools to include information about safe haven laws in their health education classes (Save Abandoned Babies Foundation, n.d.-b). Some professional groups, such as law enforcement and fire safety professionals include information on safe haven laws in their training for new professionals (Ryan et al., 2014). In general, dissemination of information about safe haven laws to the public has been deemed poor (Oberman, 2008).

Members of the news media who have reported on infants being discarded in the face of safe haven laws have declared the legislation to be unsuccessful (Buckley, 2007). One study examined illegally and legally abandoned/relinquished infants in Texas from 1996 to 2006, which was both before and after the implementation of the nation's first safe haven legislation (Pruitt, 2008). The researcher used newspaper accounts to examine infant abandonments because, as noted previously, there is no state or national system for tracking infant abandonment. The author found that during this time period, on average, the number of infant abandonments each year (7.5) was the same both before and after the implementation of the safe haven legislation and ultimately determined that safe haven laws are not particularly effective. The Save Abandoned Babies Foundation in Illinois has tallied the number of children who have been relinquished or discarded since the passage of their state's safe haven law in 2001. Between 2001 and early 2015, 103 infants have been legally relinquished to safe haven locations and 72 were illegally discarded, 37 of whom died (Save Abandoned Babies Foundation, 2015). Their tabulations show increasing numbers of infants safely and legally relinquished as opposed to being discarded. Similar statistics are cited in California (California Department of Social Services, 2013), where between 2001 and 2013, 560 infants have been safely surrendered in that state. In Los Angeles County alone, increasing numbers of infants have been safely surrendered since the passage of the state's safe haven law, as compared with the number of infants who have been discarded (Baby Safe Surrender, 2014). Figure 6.2 provides a graphical display of infants legally and illegally relinquished in Illinois and Los Angeles County from 2001 to 2013.

Conclusions about whether the law is "working" or not are questioned by those who argue that the safe relinquishment of *any* child is a success (Atwood, 2008). Still, others argue that the field has no ability to judge whether infants who are safely relinquished have been "saved" from being discarded; they might have been placed for adoption through more traditional means, where service providers would have learned about the infant's family and medical history (Deoudes, 2003; Pertman & Deoudes, 2008). Finally, scholars have argued that lacking adequate public education about the laws, it is impossible to judge their effectiveness (Oberman, 2008).

6.4.2 Too Little of the Wrong Thing, Too Late

One argument against safe haven laws is that they are a form of "crime control theater." According to this theory, crime control theater amounts to public policies which, on their face value, appear to prevent crime. They have wide public and

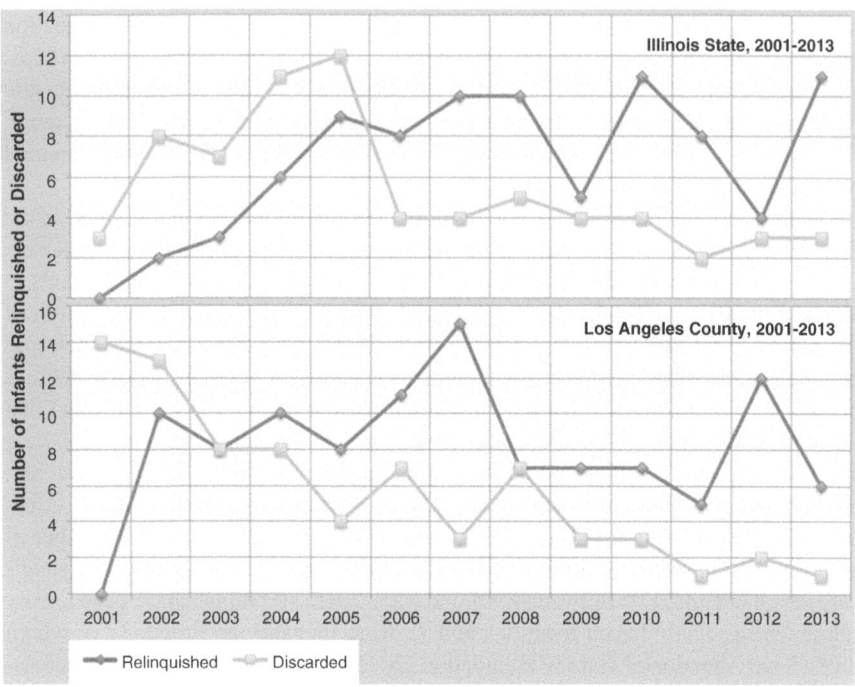

Figure 6.2 Infants Relinquished or Discarded in Illinois and Los Angeles County, 2001–2013; information comes from Save Abandoned Babies Foundation in Illinois and Baby Safe Surrender Program in Los Angeles County, California

legislative support and are generally inexpensive forms of social policy. Crime control theater theorists argue, however, that this type of policy does little to control or prevent crime, and in fact, draws resources away from crimes which are more prevalent and which are argued to be more preventable (Hammond et al., 2010). Indeed, caring for an infant who has been legally relinquished has been described as being relatively inexpensive (Save Abandoned Babies Foundation, n.d.-a). That said, safe haven laws and similar actions have also been criticized for being "too little of the wrong thing, too late." Proponents of this camp explain that in the passage of safe haven laws, states only provide options for parents who are desperate to relinquish their children, but there is little done to prevent unwanted pregnancies and few efforts to support parents who feel uneasy about their ability to care for their new children (Pollock & Hittle, 2003). The United Nations has recommended that several countries cease the use of "baby boxes" or "baby hatches," where parents can anonymously relinquish a child, and instead, recommend that government bodies focus on pregnancy prevention, counseling, and support for new parents (United Nations Committee on the Rights of the Child, 2014). As of 2014, some safe haven locations in China have been so overwhelmed with abandoned infants that they are no longer accepting new infants (Fan, 2014).

6.4.3 Marketing of Safe Haven Laws

Most of the professional literature and public attention to safe haven laws have focused on educating young, teenage parents or parents in early adulthood who are unmarried (Conover, 2000; Kopels, 2012). New England Baby Safe Haven is actively promoting the importance of using teenagers and young adults to inform the public about safe haven laws (Goss, 2014). Further marketing techniques have often focused on using prominent figures to inform young people about safe haven laws and the ability to safely and legally relinquish a child (e.g., Save Abandoned Babies Foundation uses a video featuring Steve Jobs, who was adopted as a child). There is limited research on discarded infants and even less research on their parents, in large measure because discarded infants can rarely be traced back to the parents or the individuals who abandoned them. Two of the studies of abandoned and discarded infants that I mentioned at the beginning of this chapter noted the ages of the mothers who gave up their children. The study from North Carolina, that examined discarded infants using medical examiner records from 1985 to 2000, found that 11 of the 34 infants who were discarded had parents older than 21 years; that's about one-third of the mothers (Herman-Giddens et al., 2003). Additionally, seven, or 21% of these mothers were married at the time that they discarded their infants. The Texas study of 93 infants who were abandoned (both legally and illegally) between 1996 and 2006 found that mothers' ages ranged from 15 to 40, with a mean age of 22 (Pruitt, 2008).[2] The safe haven law in Illinois was passed in 2001; between 2001 and early 2014, there have been 89 babies legally relinquished and 70 discarded, 36 of whom died. Of the information that they gathered from the mothers of these infants, the same proportion were aged 21–31 as were aged 31–41 (Ontiveros, 2014). These findings suggest that the marketing of safe haven laws to only teenagers, young adults, and first time parents may be a mistake. A recent story from the state of Wisconsin, in Textbox 6.3, illustrates the potential advisability of marketing safe haven laws to all parents expecting a new child—but not necessarily a *first* child—and to the general public at large.

Text Box 6.3
Fond du Lac, Wisconsin: Breanne Gering, a 23 year-old mother of a young child discovered that she was pregnant again and could not face the reality and financial costs of a second child. She hid the pregnancy from her family and the baby's father, and even though she knew that she was pregnant, she largely denied this fact. She was alone when she delivered a full-term infant girl in the restroom of the restaurant where she worked. She discarded the child in a dumpster, where the girl later died. Breanne had assured herself that she would return for her infant, but she did not. Later in the day she sought

(continued)

---

[2] I calculated this mean age based on descriptive information in the article.

Text Box 6.3 (continued)
medical treatment at a local hospital where she confessed to the birth and discarding her infant. Police discovered the infant girl's body later that day. Breanne was sentenced to 9 years in prison and at the writing of this chapter, is still incarcerated. She states that she did not know about safe haven laws and if she had known, she would have relinquished her infant to a safe haven location (Garbaciak, 2013).

6.4.4 Rights of "Other" Parent

Safe haven laws are primarily written with new mothers in mind. This raises important issues concerning the father of the infant. Many of the statutes are written so that a single individual, such as a parent, can relinquish an infant without supplying any additional information to the safe haven location staff. This could mean that the father of the infant may not know about the child's existence or may not know about the mother's actions (Partida, 2002). Several states have addressed this in statute by stating that attempts must be made to locate fathers prior to adoption through "family searches" conducted by child welfare agencies and the printing of public notices in newspapers (Pollock & Hittle, 2003), yet there is great variation in what state statute indicates. When mothers legally relinquish an infant and suppress all identifying information about the child, parents, and medical history, it can be very difficult to locate fathers. Legal scholars have suggested that relinquishing an infant without providing information about either parent may slow the process through which children are cleared for adoption and due process cannot be guaranteed for non-relinquishing parents (Appell, 2002b). The Child Welfare League of America recommends that before parents' rights are terminated for a given child, that the Putative Fathers Registry should be reviewed and notice of relinquishment and planned termination of parental rights should be publicized prior to termination. The League states clearly that "relinquishment by one parent should not terminate the rights of another…parent" (Pollock & Hittle, 2003, p. 25).

6.5 The Bottom Line

6.5.1 What We Know

Safe haven legislation has broad appeal to legislators and the public. The policy exists in every state in the union and it only took about a decade years for this to happen. Broadly speaking, safe haven laws have wide appeal to many different people and professions. That said, there is a large contingency which has expressed concern that safe haven laws should either be eliminated altogether (United Nations Committee on the Rights of the Child, 2014) or considered a stop-gap measure in combination with a host of pregnancy prevention or parent support efforts (Pollock & Hittle, 2003). Finally, without a federally mandated, systematic way to count and track the number of infants who are abandoned legally or illegally, we will not be able to assess the scope of the problem of infant abandonment.

Safe haven laws have provided a solution for many parents who are faced with the decision of bearing children that they do not want, cannot support, or will not raise for any number of reasons. Infants have been relinquished to safe haven locations throughout the country and there is evidence in some locations that illegal abandonments are decreasing while safe haven surrenders are increasing (California Department of Social Services, 2013; Ontiveros, 2014).

Safe haven laws are not a panacea. Infants are relinquished at safe haven locations, but very young infants continue to be abandoned, discarded, or killed throughout the country weekly (Hensley, 2013; Ranney, 2010). Safe haven laws present very real challenges to parents who are not present during surrender. Do they know about their infants? Have they turned their backs? Are they in the dark? Legal scholars have suggested that these parents, primarily fathers, cannot be guaranteed due process in the eyes of the law because of this gray area (Appell, 2002b). Child welfare professionals recommend that states step-up their efforts to better identify the unknown parents of infants who are relinquished to safe haven locations (Pollock & Hittle, 2003).

6.5.2 What Remains Unknown

The most glaring question about safe haven laws is whether they "work." The primary question as it relates to this book is whether fewer children die as a result of safe haven laws. There is presently minimal evidence that safe haven legislation results in fewer deceased children. Without safe haven laws, children who are surrendered to safe haven locations might have gone on to live with their birth parents even if those circumstances were less than ideal; they might have been raised by grandparents or other relatives; or, they might have been placed for adoption through more traditional means. We may never know whether safe haven laws are effective because methodologically speaking, it would be very difficult to resolve these unanswered questions without interviewing the individuals who relinquish the infants to inquire about their intentions. Further, what would "effective" look like? How would it be measured? Fewer discarded infants? No discarded infants? Further, we must also remember that there will always be babies who are discarded and die without knowledge to anyone but their parents. This set of factors makes it difficult and unlikely that we would ever know the true effectiveness of safe haven laws.

Children continue to be killed and discarded or discarded and die even though safe haven laws are in place. This is where the need for multiple approaches to prevent unwanted pregnancy and to provide parent support comes into play. Safe haven laws provide a legitimate resource for parents who are thinking reasonably and rationally in the face of an unwanted child. For those who are in a state of emotional distress or denial, safe haven laws may not even enter the picture. At this time, those are the parents that the field has not yet figured out how to reach.

The public awareness and knowledge of safe haven laws is generally unknown. Most safe haven laws were passed without adequate funding for implementation, including training, public education, or outreach (Oberman, 2008). Safe haven laws cannot be declared as a success or failure if we do not know how much of the public or providers know about them. This speaks to the need for broader public education among professionals working with expecting parents and broad scale public education throughout communities. States could also take a page from Illinois, which now requires that information about safe haven relinquishment be implemented into the high school curriculum (Save Abandoned Babies Foundation, n.d.-b). Such an approach could be taken in other states by legislating where information is distributed and what professional groups must receive training.

References

Abandoned Infants Assistance Act, Pub. L. No. 100–505 (1988 October 18).
Appell, A. R. (2002a). Safe havens to abandon babies, Part I: The law. *Adoption Quarterly, 5*(4), 59–68.
Appell, A. R. (2002b). Safe havens to abandon babies, Part III: The effects. *Adoption Quarterly, 6*(2), 67–76.
Atwood, T. C. (2008). Comment: National Council for Adoption's response to the Texas Safe Haven study. *Child Maltreatment, 13*(1), 96–97. doi:10.1177/1077559507310367.
Baby left overnight in woods; mother held (2014, April 21). *The News & Record*. Retrieved from http://www.sovanow.com/index.php?/news/article/baby_left_overnight_in_woods_mother_held/
Baby Safe Surrender. (2014). *About the baby safe surrender program*. Retrieved June 13, 2014, from http://babysafela.org/about/
Buckley, C. (2007). Safe-haven laws fail to end discarding of babies. *New York Times*. Retrieved from http://www.nytimes.com/2007/01/13/nyregion/13babies.html?pagewanted=all&_r=0
California Department of Social Services. (2013). *Safely surrendered baby law*. Retrieved June 13, 2014, from http://www.babysafe.ca.gov/
Carter, T. F. (2013, November 5). Secret Safe Place for Newborns celebrates 15 years of success. *AL.com*. Retrieved from http://blog.al.com/pr-community-news/2013/11/the_secret_safe_place_for_newb.html
Child Welfare Information Gateway. (2010). *"Infant safe haven laws" summary of state laws*. Retrieved January 14, 2015, from http://www.childwelfare.gov/systemwide/laws_policies/statutes/safehaven.pdf
Conover, M. (2000, July 6). Teens need to be educated about baby 'safe haven' law. *Indianapolis Star*, p. W2.
Curran, L., & Pletrzak, J. (2001, Spring). AIA Programs: Yesterday, today, and tomorrow. *The Source: The National Abandoned Infants Assistance Resource Center*. Retrieved June 9, 2014, Spring, from http://aia.berkeley.edu/media/pdf/10_year_retrospective_spring_2001.pdf

References

D.C. Council OKs newborn safe haven. (2009, April 8). *The Washington Times*. Retrieved from http://www.washingtontimes.com/news/2009/apr/08/council-approves-safe-haven-for-babies/

Deoudes, G. (2003). *Unintended consequences: "Safe haven" laws are causing problems, not solving them*. New York, NY: The Donaldson Adoption Institute.

Domash, S. F., Gallucci, J., & Twarowski, C. (2010, October 14). *Inside Tim Jaccard's Children of Hope and baby safe haven crusade*. Long Island Press. Retrieved from http://archive.longislandpress.com/2010/10/14/inside-tim-jaccards-children-of-hope-and-baby-safe-haven-crusade/

Douglas, E. M. (2006). *State-level predictors of divorce-related public policy*. Paper presented at the 6th Annual state politics and policy conference, Lubbock, TX.

Douglas, E. M., & Mohn, B. L. (2014). *Safe haven legislation in the United States: An exploratory analysis*. Paper presented at the Policy conference 2.0, Austin, TX. http://sites.stedwards.edu/policyconference2/

Fan, W. (2014, June 24). 'Safe haven' overwhelmed with abandoned babies. *China News Service*. Retrieved from http://www.ecns.cn/2014/06-24/120579.shtml

Garbaciak, J. (2013, November 19). Mother who left baby in dumpster talks to WISN 12 News about why she did it. *WISN12 ABC*. Retrieved from http://www.wisn.com/news/mother-who-left-baby-in-dumpster-talks-to-wisn-12-news-about-why-she-did-it/-/9373668/23039766/-/o5l81h/-/index.html#ixzz343bDxJIp

Goss, C. (2014, July 16). Dalhart pushes for education on baby safe haven laws. *ConnectAmarillo.com*. Retrieved from http://www.connectamarillo.com/news/story.aspx?id=1071149#.U8hVXvldU6w

Hammond, M., Miller, M. K., & Griffin, T. (2010). Safe haven laws as crime control theater. *Child Abuse & Neglect, 34*(7), 545–552.

Hensley, J. J. (2013, October 12). Many remain unaware of baby safe haven laws. *USA Today*. Retrieved from http://www.usatoday.com/story/news/nation/2013/10/12/advocates-struggle-to-raise-awareness-of-baby-safe-haven-laws/2973177/

Herman-Giddens, M. E., Smith, J. B., Mittal, M., Carlson, M., & Butts, J. D. (2003). Newborns killed or left to die by a parent: A population-based study. *JAMA, 289*(11), 1425–1429.

Kertzer, D. I. (1991). Gender ideology and infant abandonment in nineteenth-century Italy. *The Journal of Interdisciplinary History, 22*(1), 1–25. doi:10.2307/204563.

Kopels, S. (2012). Safe haven laws and school social work. *School Social Work Journal, 36*(2), 27–43.

McKee, G. R. (2006). *Why mothers kill: A forensic psychologist's casebook*. New York, NY: Oxford University Press.

Meyer, C., Oberman, M., & Rone, M. (2001). *Mothers who kill their children: Understanding the acts of moms from Susan Smith to the "prom mom"*. New York, NY: New York University Press.

Mondo, M. (2014, January 15). Mom said she strangled newborn, watched him die. *San Antonio Express News*. Retrieved from http://www.mysanantonio.com/news/local/article/Mom-said-she-strangled-newborn-watched-him-die-5144862.php

National Abandoned Infants Assistance Resource Center. (2005, December). *Boarder babies, abandoned infants, and discarded infants*. Retrieved June 9, 2014, from http://aia.berkeley.edu/media/pdf/abandoned_infant_fact_sheet_2005.pdf

National Safe Haven Alliance. (n.d.). *Baby safe haven – Abandoned infant protection laws*. Retrieved January 4, 2015, from http://www.nationalsafehavenalliance.org/law.php

Oberman, M. (2008). Comment: Infant abandonment in Texas. *Child Maltreatment, 13*(1), 94–95. doi:10.1177/1077559507310044.

Ontiveros, S. (2014, February 14). Pass the word, Illinois' safe haven law works. *Chicago Sun-Times*. Retrieved from http://www.suntimes.com/news/ontiveros/25546348-452/pass-the-word-illinois-safe-haven-law-works.html#.U5oQ8vldU6w

Partida, A. L. (2002). The case for 'safe haven' laws: Choosing the lesser of two evils in a disposable society. *New England Journal on Criminal & Civil Confinement, 28*, 61–61.

Patterson, J. (2014, May 7). Dinwiddie mother walks free after newborn drowns in toilet. *CBS6*. Retrieved from http://wtvr.com/2014/05/07/dinwiddie-mother-accused-of-murdering--newborn-walks-free/comment-page-1/

Pertman, A., & Deoudes, G. (2008). Comment: Evan B. Donaldson Adoption Institute response. *Child Maltreatment, 13*(1), 98–100. doi:10.1177/1077559507310368.

Pollock, K., & Hittle, L. (2003). *Baby abandonment: The role of child welfare systems.* Retrieved from http://66.227.70.18/programs/baby/babymonographintro.pdf

Pruitt, S. L. (2008). The number of illegally abandoned and legally surrendered newborns in the state of Texas, estimated from news stories, 1996–2006. *Child Maltreatment, 13*(1), 89–93.

Rafferty, A. (2013, February 28). Hoping for a 'fresh start,' mother abandons child in woods. *NBC News*. Retrieved from http://usnews.nbcnews.com/_news/2013/02/28/17137418-hoping-for-a-fresh-start-mother-abandons-child-in-woods?lite

Ranney, D. (2010, July 14). Tragedies continue but safe haven law remains unused. *Kansas Health Institute*. Retrieved from http://www.khi.org/news/2010/jul/14/tragedies-continue-safe-haven-law-remains-unused/

Recognizing Mobile County district attorney John Tyson and his work in creating the Alabama Secret Safe Place program, U.S. House of Representatives E1615 (2008).

Ryan, M., Caputo, N. D., & Berrett, O. M. (2014). Safe Haven Laws: Lack of awareness, misinformation, and shortfalls in resident education. *The American Journal of Emergency Medicine, 32*(1), 98–100. doi:10.1016/j.ajem.2013.10.015.

Save Abandoned Babies Foundation. (2015). *Time line & facts.* Chicago, IL: Save Abandoned Babies Foundation.

Save Abandoned Babies Foundation. (n.d.-a). *Frequently asked questions.* Retrieved January 20, 2015, from http://www.saveabandonedbabies.org/resources/FAQ/

Save Abandoned Babies Foundation. (n.d.-b). *Safe haven law teacher's kit.* Retrieved June 13, 2014, from http://www.saveabandonedbabies.org/resources/teaching_tools/posters/teacher_kit.pdf

Tebo, M. G. (2001). Texas Idea Takes Off. *ABA Journal, 87*(9), 30.

Tilly, L. A., Fuchs, R. G., Kertzer, D. I., & Ransel, D. L. (1992). Child abandonment in European history:A symposium. *Journal of Family History, 17*(1), 1–23. doi:10.1177/036319909201700101.

U.S. Department of Health & Human Services. (1994). *Children's Bureau: Report to the Congress: National estimates on the number of boarder babies, the cost of their care, and the number of abandonment infants.* Washington, DC: U.S. Department of Health & Human Services.

U.S. Department of Health & Human Services. (1998). *1998 National estimates of the number of boarder babies, abandoned infants and discarded infants.* Washington, DC. Retrieved from https://www.ncjrs.gov/pdffiles1/Photocopy/191716NCJRS.pdf

United Nations Committee on the Rights of the Child. (2014). *Concluding observations on the combined fourth and fifth periodic reports of the Russian Federation* (CRC/C/RUS/CO/4-5). Geneva, Switzerland: United Nations. Retrieved from http://www.refworld.org/docid/52f89e2b4.html

Chapter 7
Criminal Justice and Legal Reforms in Response to Fatal Child Maltreatment

The challenges associated with the investigation, prosecution, and convictions in cases of child abuse and neglect have been well documented (Cross, Walsh, Simone, & Jones, 2003). There is limited evidence, victims are young and may be less reliable than older children, victims do not always come forward, and there is stigma concerning who is capable of harming a child. Many of these same problems exist in the prosecution in cases of fatal child maltreatment. One of the main difficulties have been that when law enforcement encounters a deceased child, they often fail to conduct investigations and collect evidence in a manner that is consistent with standards for basic criminal investigations (Commonwealth of Virginia Department for Children, 1990). There are also obstacles with prosecution because of insufficient evidence in maltreatment-related homicides. Therefore, it is legally difficult to charge perpetrators with serious crimes. Instead, perpetrators are often charged with endangering the welfare of a child or manslaughter. Finally, even if sufficient evidence is collected, and the perpetrators are charged with a crime, it can be difficult to convince a jury that parents and other caregivers could use so much violence or treat a child with such callous disregard as to end a child's life (Griffin, 2004).

Almost two decades ago, the problems associated with fatal child maltreatment and criminal justice were documented in a report issued by the U.S. Department of Health & Human Services, called "A Nation's Shame" (United States Advisory Board on Child Abuse and Neglect, 1995). Despite multiple efforts to address these problems, many of the issues outlined in that report remain. This is the focus of the current chapter.

7.1 The Scope of the Problem

7.1.1 Problems with Investigations

Literature beginning in the 1990s noted that first responders to child death scenes often failed to consider that children's deaths could be due to abuse and neglect. As a result, these first responders commonly did not collect sufficient evidence from the scene and did not interview family members and caregivers. When maltreatment was eventually suspected, it became difficult to pursue criminal charges due to lack of sufficient evidence. A 1990 report by the Commonwealth of Virginia, Department of Children (1990) determined that the primary reason why perpetrators of fatal child maltreatment were not charged and/or convicted of harsh sentences was the result of poor investigative practices on the part of law enforcement. The committee that wrote this report cited numerous problems, including a lack of evidence, insufficient evidence that would not be accepted by the court, or poorly conducted investigations. These problems were also noted by the United States Advisory Board on Child Abuse and Neglect (1995) in the mid-1990s.

Limitations in the practices around child death investigations are not specific to law enforcement. For decades now, the literature on fatal child maltreatment has noted the under-ascertainment, or under-recognition by medical examiners of deaths due to abuse and neglect (see Chapter 2) (Crume, DiGuiseppi, Byers, Sirotnak, & Garrett, 2002; Ewigman, Kivlahan, & Land, 1993; Gessner, Moore, Hamilton, & Muth, 2004; Herman-Giddens et al., 1999; Klevens & Leeb, 2010; Soerdjbalie-Maikoe, Bilo, van den Akker, & Maes, 2010). This under-recognition has been linked to a number of reasons: failing to suspect child abuse or neglect as a potential cause, lack of knowledge concerning abuse and neglect deaths, mistaking a maltreatment case for an unintended injury, accident, or sudden infant death syndrome/sudden unexplained infant death syndrome (SIDS/SUDS), restrictions of standardized coding for deaths, and differences of opinion regarding what constitutes maltreatment (Crume et al., 2002; Emery, 1993; Herman-Giddens et al., 1999; Levene & Bacon, 2004).

The best example of this latter issue—what constitutes abuse or neglect—is the current debate over whether children who die as a result of co-sleeping or bed-sharing with family members or pets die from neglect (or abuse) and whether their deaths are ruled as accidental. The possible factors to consider are endless: What if child protective services had instructed the parents not to co-sleep with their children? Or, what if the parents are from a culture or country where co-sleeping is routinely and primarily safely practiced? What if the parents were intoxicated or obese? What if the child died as a result of co-sleeping but suffered from abuse or neglect prior to death? What if the child had no safe sleeping environment in the home (Kim, Shapiro-Mendoza, Chu, Camperlengo, & Anderson, 2012)? In Wisconsin an intoxicated parent smothered his infant and was convicted of felony child neglect. In response, a state legislator drafted a new bill that would hold all intoxicated parents of a sleeping-related infant/child death criminally responsible

7.1 The Scope of the Problem

(Causey, 2012; Davis & Polcyn, 2014). Meanwhile, professionals whose focus is to promote breastfeeding have recently argued that telling parents to refrain from co-sleeping in beds has contributed to parents co-sleeping with their infants on couches or recliners, which have been linked to more infant deaths (Bartick, 2014). These are issues that have not been resolved and continue to be debated today (Huyer, 2014; M. D. Overpeck, Personal communication, December 10, 2013; Shapiro-Mendoza, Camperlengo, Kim, & Covington, 2012).

In addition to the problems already noted, in homes where chronic abuse and/or neglect is present, it can be difficult to determine who is ultimately responsible for a child's death (Griffin, 2004; Holmgren, 2001). Text Box 7.1 documents the brutal death of 6-month-old Brianna Lopez, who was killed in New Mexico by her father and uncle. They raped her and physically threw her around their home the night before she died; her mother was present for these abusive and criminal acts, but did not intervene. After death, medical examiners found Brianna's body was marked with numerous injuries in various stages of healing. In this particular instance, all three caretakers were held responsible for the child's death, but it is unclear who was ultimately responsible (Staley, 2014).

Text Box 7.1
"Baby Brianna was not quite 6-months old when she died, July 19, 2002. The night before, her father, Andrew Walters, and uncle, Steven Lopez, reportedly threw the small child around their house and raped her. Her mother, Stephanie Lopez, let it happen, authorities said. Baby Brianna's tiny body had bite marks, broken bones and evidence that she was healing from previous injuries. Stephanie Lopez was sentenced to 27 years for counts of negligent child abuse resulting in death, and child abuse. But because of credit for time served, she can be paroled after 13.5 years. Walters, 32, and Steven Lopez, 31, had more serious convictions so they won't be eligible for release from prison till 2042 and 2039, respectively…" (Staley, 2014).

7.1.2 Limited Charges

Historically speaking, limits on the definitions of murder have caused difficulties in prosecuting perpetrators of child abuse and neglect-related deaths. Cases of fatal child maltreatment do not generally involve premeditation or intent to cause death—provisions that are traditionally part of the legal definition of murder (Stewart, 1990). Instead, children are usually killed in the heat of the moment, through careless actions as part of discipline or lashing out in anger; or, children die as a result of parental omission, such as failing to supervise children in life-threatening situations or failing to give medical care (see Chapter 2). As a result, charges have often been reduced to manslaughter or a lesser charge (Stewart, 1990), such as endangering the welfare of a child (Bendetowies, 1990).

7.1.3 Problems Persist into the Courtroom

Even if the obstacles already addressed were adequately handled, problems can mount in the courtroom. Anecdotal evidence suggests that jurors can be reluctant to believe that a parent, relative, or caregiver would hurt his or her own child (Bendetowies, 1990; Rainey & Greer, 1994; United States Advisory Board on Child Abuse and Neglect, 1995). For example, in Pennsylvania in 2014, a toddler was killed by her mother when the mother squeezed the child so hard that it caused internal injuries and the child bled to death. A neighbor responded to the death and arrest of the mother by saying: "That's [the child's] mom…[she] gave birth to [her]…why would she do something like that to her own kid?" (Hughes, 2014). Similarly, also in 2014, a father in the state of Georgia was accused of purposely leaving his toddler in a hot car for 7 hours, as a means to kill him. Some members of the public rallied around the father, putting pressure on law enforcement to drop the charges, with statements such as: "These were very loving parents who are devastated. Justin [the father] already has to live with a punishment worse than death" (Parry, 2014). The emotional suffering of the parents is an often-cited reason for not wanting to pursue a criminal case against individuals responsible for their children's deaths (Collins, 2006). Thus, it can be difficult to achieve a successful criminal conviction, even with what may otherwise be considered sufficient evidence.

All parents have been "less than perfect" at some point. Prosecutors have speculated that jurors who are also parents can sometimes identify with individuals on the stand, when they remember a time when they got angrier at their children than they would have liked or grabbed or spanked them harder than they had intended (Mills & Kiernan, 1998). On the opposite end of the spectrum, jurors might remember when they turned away from their child, didn't notice their child crossing a busy street, left their infant in the car when they quickly ran inside a convenience store, or when they accidentally fell asleep while their toddler roamed the house unsupervised. Sometimes children are killed by single incidences of rage or negligence and most parents can remember single instances when they were "less than" optimum parents.

7.2 Innovative Approaches at Multiple Levels

7.2.1 Changes in Investigative Techniques

One of the most significant changes made in the criminal justice system concerns the way investigations of child fatalities are handled, from first responders all the way to the medical examiner. Discussions concerning this element of criminal justice work began in the 1970s (Rollins & Nickerson, 1978) and continued for the next several decades, increasingly being taken on by government agencies and professional associations (American Prosecutors Research Institute, 1994; Illinois

Dept of Children and Family Services, 1986; Kaplan & Granik, 1991; Sirotnak & Brittain, 2006; U. S. Department of Justice, 2000; Walsh, 2005; Washoe County Child Death Review Team, n.d.; Westveer, 1997).

Guidebooks regarding how to investigate sudden or unexplained deaths of infants walk first responders through the steps that they need to take in order to ensure that investigations on young victims are carried out appropriately and that adequate evidence is collected at the scene. The guidebook from the U.S. Centers for Disease Control and Prevention tries to prepare first responders for the unique circumstances of infant deaths by noting: "Infant death scenes can become crowded with emotional family members and witnesses" (Hanzlick, Jentzen, & Clark, 2007, p. 3). This note of caution reflects how easy it can be for first responders to become distracted by emotion and disregard infant death scenes as possible crime scenes (Stanton & Simpson, 2001).

The most comprehensive guidebook that has been written about investigating child deaths was published by the Department of Justice (Walsh, 2005). In this practical guide, Walsh explains not only how to approach a child's death from an investigatory point of view, but why such an approach is necessary and how these investigations differ from other homicides. For example, there are likely few witnesses to the crime, because most children die in their homes in the company of the caregivers who are likely responsible for their deaths. Additionally, children are rarely killed with weapons that are traditionally used in other homicides, such as firearms or knives. Instead, children are most likely to be killed with a caregiver's hands and feet. Injuries are likely to result from shaking, scalding water, neglectful supervision, and other such acts carried out by maltreating families. The motives for child deaths are usually distinct from those in other homicides. Instead of a child's death being planned or in response to jealously or during the act of another crime, children are often killed when parental discipline gets "out of control" or in response to frustration with a child. Like the guidebook by the U.S. Centers for Disease Control and Prevention, this book lays out instructions for every stage of the investigation. It provides a rationale for why it is important to cooperate with child protective services as these professionals may be able to help to determine if maltreatment was present and may be able to protect surviving siblings in a case where abuse or neglect are involved.

Beginning in the 1970s, there have been initiatives by law enforcement agencies, attorneys general, district attorneys, and professional associations to improve accuracy in the investigations of cases of fatal child maltreatment (San Diego County Office of the District Attorney, 1977). The purpose of these trainings has been to educate law enforcement and attorneys about the differences between sudden infant death syndrome and deaths caused by maltreatment, how to gather adequate evidence at the scene, interview caregivers, and put together a solid legal case that will stand up in court (Dallas Police Department, 1994; Garstang & Sidebotham, 2008).

7.2.2 Legal Responses to Increase Penalties for Child Abuse and Neglect Deaths

As a nation, the United States started to pay closer attention to death by abuse and neglect in the 1980s–1990s. During this time, even when evidence showed that a crime had been committed and a body of jurors willing to consider conviction, prosecutors' hands were tied because the nature of fatal child maltreatment did not allow for the prosecution of murder, manslaughter, and so forth. Instead, prosecutors had to charge perpetrators with less serious crimes, such as endangering the welfare of a child (Stewart, 1990). State legislatures began to address this issue by passing new legislation or modifying existing legislation that would allow for harsher crimes to be prosecuted and more serious penalties to be applied when a child died as a result of abuse or neglect (Bendetowies, 1990; Vollrath, 2011). This movement toward child-specific homicide statutes has received limited attention in professional publications, even though it has been addressed at the legislative level by many states (National Center for the Prosecution of Child Abuse, 2013). The issue of criminal sentencing in cases of fatal child maltreatment has most often been handled by law journals, advocacy organizations, or government-affiliated teams (such as child death review teams—see Chapter 5).

Phipps (1999) has addressed child homicide statutes in a more comprehensive manner than any other scholar. He describes how states have handled the legal quandary concerning the harsher conviction and sentencing of penalties for perpetrating fatal child maltreatment through two primary methods, both of which are based on the age of the victim. In the first method, the killing of a child by abuse or neglect is reclassified as a homicide, even if the circumstances of the victim's death would not have met the criteria for homicide if the victim were an adult. In the second method, the classification of the crime itself does not change; instead, the sentence that is imposed is harsher because the victim was a child. Most of these laws were passed in the mid-to-late 1990s.

There are three defining characteristics of child homicide statutes (Phipps, 1999). First, the statute must be a homicide statute. This is important because there are other legal ways to increase the penalty for killing a child, without convicting the perpetrator of the crime of homicide. Second, a homicide statute punishes an individual for killing a child while that individual was perpetrating child maltreatment against the child. Third, child homicide statutes do not require evidence that the perpetrator intended to kill a child with his or her actions or inactions.

The statutes themselves generally fall into two categories (Phipps, 1999). First is a *homicide by abuse* statute, which is a separate offense and unrelated to other homicide provisions. These types of statutes generally include three elements: (1) a perpetrator is engaged in maltreating a child and then kills that child by that maltreatment, (2) the perpetrator demonstrates extreme indifference to the worth of human life, and (3) the victim is under an age which is considered by the state to be especially vulnerable. South Carolina's child homicide statute, for example, addresses all of these components.

7.2 Innovative Approaches at Multiple Levels

South Carolina. (A) A person is guilty of homicide by child abuse if the person: (1) causes the death of a child under the age of eleven while committing child abuse or neglect, and the death occurs under circumstances manifesting an extreme indifference to human life; or (2) knowingly aids and abets another person to commit child abuse or neglect, and the child abuse or neglect results in the death of a child under the age of eleven.

(B) For purposes of this section, the following definitions apply: (1) "child abuse or neglect" means an act or omission by any person which causes harm to the child's physical health or welfare; (2) "harm" to a child's health or welfare occurs when a person: (a) inflicts or allows to be inflicted upon the child physical injury, including injuries sustained as a result of excessive corporal punishment; (b) fails to supply the child with adequate food, clothing, shelter, or health care, and the failure to do so causes a physical injury or condition resulting in death; or (c) abandons the child resulting in the child's death.

(C) Homicide by child abuse is a felony and a person who is convicted of or pleads guilty to homicide by child abuse: (1)...may be imprisoned for life or no less than a term of twenty years; or (2)...must be imprisoned for a term not exceeding twenty years nor less than ten years.

(D) In sentencing...the judge must consider any aggravating circumstances including, but not limited to, a defendant's past pattern of child abuse or neglect of a child under the age of eleven, and any mitigating circumstances; however, a child's crying does not constitute provocation so as to be considered a mitigating circumstance. (South Carolina Code Annotated, §16-3-85)

The second type of child homicide statute is a *felony murder statute*, which includes child maltreatment as a type of felony that could result in homicide. These statutes tend to be less complex because they simply connect the killing of a child while simultaneously committing felony child maltreatment against the child. Maryland is one example of this type of child homicide statute.

Maryland. Child abuse in the first degree: (b) (1) A parent, family member, household member, or other person who has permanent or temporary care or custody or responsibility for the supervision of a minor may not cause abuse to the minor that: (i) results in the death of the minor...(2) Except as provided in subsection (c) of this section, a person who violates paragraph (1) of this subsection is guilty of the felony of child abuse in the first degree and on conviction is subject to...imprisonment not exceeding 40 years. (Maryland Code Annotated Criminal Law §3-601)

Finally, there are additional ways to increase the penalties for taking a child's life by abuse or neglect, without passing a child homicide statute. These types of laws do not address the type of offense that was committed or the charges brought against the perpetrator. Instead, they only address the length of the penalty that is applied after conviction for a criminal offense that caused a child's death. Maine, for example, has a law that states that in murder cases where the victim was a child, the age of the child can be a determining factor when the judge is deciding sentencing.

Maine. In setting the length of imprisonment [for murder], if the victim is a child who had not in fact attained the age of 6 years at the time the crime was committed...a court shall assign special weight to this objective fact in determining the...sentence. (Maine Revised Statute Annotated Title 17-A, §1251)

7.2.3 Special Legal Reforms in Response to Religiously-Motivated Medical Child Maltreatment Fatalities

There have been substantive changes in one area of child protection and criminal codes that have resulted in increased prosecution, conviction, and penalties for individuals who are responsible for children's deaths. These are in the area of religiously-motivated medical child maltreatment, which I first introduced in Chapter 2. The public often scorns parents who, because of their religious beliefs, allow their children to die without medical treatment. However, public policies throughout the United States provide exemptions to medical mandates because of religious beliefs. These laws originate with the 1974 Child Abuse Prevention and Treatment Act (CAPTA). This legislation shaped the then-developing field of child welfare, and mandated all states to adopt religious-based exemptions to charges or substantiations of child maltreatment. Federal funding for states' child welfare programs was contingent on the adoption of such language and it affected both civil and criminal laws. Although this language was repealed from federal law in 1983, states had already adopted the provisions that were formerly mandated for almost a decade, and there wasn't a strong enough backlash against "religious shield" laws to overturn them. In the 1996 re-authorization of CAPTA, non-mandatory language concerning religious-exemptions was reintroduced into the law, stating that failure to provide medical care because of religious beliefs would not constitute maltreatment (Swan, 1997). That provision remained through the 2010 reauthorization as well (Swan, 2010): "Nothing in this act shall be construed as establishing a Federal requirement that a parent or legal guardian provide a child any medical service or treatment against the religious beliefs of the parent or legal guardian" ("Child Abuse Prevention and Treatment Act," 1996, §113).

Since 1975, approximately 400 child deaths associated with religious-based medical neglect in the United States have been documented (personal communication with R. Swan, July 30, 2014). Children's Healthcare Is a Legal Duty (CHILD) is a nonprofit organization that works to overturn religious shield laws with regard to the maltreatment of children. This organization reports that one cemetery that is used in Idaho by the Followers of Christ, which is a faith-healing sect, has 553 graves and over 30% of those graves are for deceased children and stillbirths. Overall in Idaho only 3.37% of all deaths occur to children, which is vastly lower than what was found in this one "sample" of deceased members of Followers of Christ (Children's Healthcare Is a Legal Duty, 2014). Faith-healing has increasingly been the subject of media attention (Biema, 1998; Margolick, 1990; Tilkin, 2013). Research has shown that the majority of children's deaths that are associated with religiously-motivated medical neglect have been extremely painful to the child victims and could have been prevented with standard medical treatment (Asser & Swan, 1998). Text Boxes 7.2 and 7.3 provide two examples of religiously-motivated medical child neglect that were prosecuted in the courts; examples are taken from the website of CHILD.

Text Box 7.2
"In 1986, Robyn Twitchell, age 2, who lived near Boston, died of peritonitis and a twisted bowel after a five-day illness. It began with...screaming and vomiting. [On day two]...his parents...called the Christian Science church... which assured them ...[of their] right to use Christian Science treatment instead of medical treatment. On...day four, a church nurse recorded: 'Child listless at times, rejecting all food, moaning in pain, three wounds on thigh.' The nurse...and his mother...force-fed him...every half hour. On the fifth day, he was vomiting 'a brown, foul-smelling substance.' Neighbors closed their bedroom window so they would not hear [Robyn's] screams. At the Twitchells' trial, a Christian Science practitioner testified that she...achieved a complete healing of Robyn and that he had run around...chasing his...cat 15 minutes before he died. Rigor mortis had set in before the parents called 911. The parents were convicted of manslaughter in 1990...[which was] overturned...on a technicality, but also ruled that parents had a legal duty to provide necessary medical care for their children regardless of their religious beliefs."

Text Box 7.3
"In 1998 two-year-old Harrison Johnson was stung 432 times by wasps while the family was visiting church friends in Tampa, Florida. His parents asked neighborhood children and fellow church members to pray for him, but did not call for medical help until more than 7 hours after the attack. Six minutes after the 911 call, the EMT's arrived to find the toddler without a pulse and not breathing. His pupils were fixed and dilated. His parents [said] the boy had been unresponsive for 30 to 45 minutes. An Orlando pediatrician [said] that the toddler would likely have displayed alarming symptoms. He would have been crying and in great pain until he slipped into shock. His lungs would have filled with fluid. His parents belong to a group called The Fellowship, which reportedly shuns all medical care on grounds that doctors practice witchcraft. The Johnsons were charged with felony child abuse. The judge, however, instructed the jury that the state must prove that the parents willfully or intentionally caused the harm to the child. The jury acquitted."

Some argue that denying healthcare to children on religious grounds denies a particular class of children rights that are enjoyed by all other children in the United States (Swan, 1998), thus making exemptions, in the eyes of some legal professionals, unconstitutional (Lamparello, 2001). In fact, there have been legal rulings where the rights of children were favored over the rights of their parents ("In re: Clark," 1962; "Prince v. Massachusetts," 1944). Still others have drawn attention to countries such as Canada and some in the European Union, which do not permit religious exemptions to children's healthcare. Parents are legally obligated to seek medical attention for children regardless of religious doctrine (Hamilton, 2003; Scolnick, 1990).

Since the late 1980s, the Committee of Bioethics of the American Academy of Pediatrics has called for a repeal of religious-based exemptions to mandates for children's healthcare (American Academy of Pediatrics, 1988, 1997) and in 2003 some 30 U.S. organizations that work to prevent child maltreatment, unsuccessfully called for Congress to lift the religious shield in CAPTA (Children's Healthcare Is a Legal Duty, n.d.-b). One study found that the general public in the state of Florida also believed that medical professionals should override parents' desires concerning religious beliefs around medical care. They were less enthusiastic about parents being criminally prosecuted for failing to provide medical treatment because of religious reasons, however (Hartog, Freeman, Kubilis, & Janowski, 1999).

Nevertheless, there have been increases in the numbers of parents who have been criminally prosecuted for allowing their children to die because of failure to provide medical care based on religious beliefs. This increase is largely attributed to Rita Swan, a former Christian Scientist who allowed her 18-month-old son to die in the 1970s because of failing to provide medical care. After her son's death she quickly became a pioneer in overturning religious shield laws throughout the country. Her story and the work that she has accomplished through her organization, CHILD, is well documented in the recent trade book, *In the Name of God: The True Story of the Fight to Save Children from Faith-Healing Homicide* (Stauth, 2013). Since 1990, Swan has helped to repeal religious exemptions that permit parents to withhold medical treatment because of religious preferences in Arizona, Colorado, Delaware, Hawaii, Maryland, Massachusetts, Minnesota, North Carolina, Rhode Island, Oregon, and South Dakota (Children's Healthcare Is a Legal Duty, n.d.-a), but many such laws remain throughout the United States.

7.3 Are Criminal Penalties Increasing?

The idea of increased penalties for fatal maltreatment has been on the policy table in every state in the Union in some form for two to three decades. In fact, most states have implemented some form of legislation that makes it possible to more harshly punish individuals who kill a child while perpetrating abuse or neglect (National Center for the Prosecution of Child Abuse, 2013; Phipps, 1999). As is the case with many social policy reforms (D'Andrade & Berrick, 2006; Douglas, 2006; Mazzola, Mohiddin, Ward, & Holdsworth, 2013; Sanchez, Nock, Wright, Pardee, & Ionescu, 2001), we don't know whether these policy changes have been implemented in practice. There has been limited research in this area and few attempts to track the criminal justice outcomes in cases of fatal maltreatment. Furthermore, there have been no attempts to link changes in policy to criminal justice outcomes.

7.3 Are Criminal Penalties Increasing?

Research shows that there are few central or ongoing efforts to examine the criminal justice outcomes of cases of fatal child maltreatment. Research I conducted in the late 1990s revealed that a handful of states and jurisdictions had compiled this information from a variety of sources, including child death review teams, offices of district attorneys/attorneys general, newspaper accounts, and publications in peer-reviewed sources (Douglas, 1999). In total, I compiled information from eight different locations: Los Angeles County in California, Dallas County in Texas, the State of Florida, North Carolina, Maine, selected counties in Colorado, the city of Chicago in Illinois, and a children's hospital in Dayton, Ohio (Hicks & Gaughan, 1995). There was significant variation in what was reported. Some locations reported on the nature of convictions, others reported on the penalties imposed; others reported on both. The overarching theme among all of the sources of data was that perpetrators were convicted of crimes that had less severe penalties, such as endangering the welfare of a child, knowing/reckless child abuse, involuntary manslaughter, and criminally negligent homicide. Many times these convictions or guilty pleas were not accompanied by jail time, only probation. In addition, there were also many instances when criminal charges were never brought against a perpetrator for the death of a child.

Current research shows that information on the criminal justice outcomes of fatal child maltreatment remains just as fragmented today. Information is sporadically available by all of the same sources that I used about 15 years ago: child death review team reports, advocacy organizations, state offices on child maltreatment or child and families, peer-reviewed sources, and exposés in the media. These sources indicate that there is potentially greater variation today in how cases of fatal maltreatment are handled by the criminal justice system.

The North Carolina Child Advocacy Institute (2005) examined 23 cases, with 24 perpetrators, of fatal child abuse in North Carolina in 1998. The criminal convictions for the perpetrators are not indicated in the report, only their criminal justice penalties, which are noted here:

- 8 Never changed/No jail time
- 3 Received less than 2 years
- 2 Received 2–5 years
- 2 Received 5–10 years
- 5 Received 10–25 years
- 2 Received 40 years
- 2 Received life sentences

The National Center for the Review and Prevention of Child Deaths (n.d.) provides guidelines for what child death review teams should include in their annual reports. There are currently no recommendations pertaining to the criminal justice outcomes of perpetrators of fatal child maltreatment. Nevertheless, historically a handful of child death review teams, including those in Maine, North Carolina, and Los Angeles County, have published statistics on the criminal justice outcomes of maltreatment-related deaths. The latest report from the Los Angeles County child death review team describes both the legal convictions and penalties for child homicides that occurred between 2004 and 2011; those outcomes are summarized in Table 7.1 (Inter-Agency on Child Abuse and Neglect, 2012). A small proportion of

Table 7.1 Criminal Dispositions of Child Homicides by Parent, Caretaker, or Family Member

Criminal Disposition	Number of Cases	Percent of Cases
Pending at time of publication	59	23.7
Conviction, sentencing pending	3	1.2
Mental competency hearing pending	4	1.6
Arrest warrant issued	3	1.2
Case dismissed	6	2.4
Found not guilty	2	0.8
Sentenced to probation	11	4.4
Sentenced to jail time:		0.0
• 1 year	7	2.8
• 1–3 years	17	6.8
• 4–5 years	10	4.0
• 6–10 years	29	11.6
• 11–19 years	46	18.5
• 10 years-Life	44	17.7
• Life	8	3.2
Total	249	100%

Adapted from Inter-Agency on Child Abuse and Neglect (2012). Child death review team report 2012: Report compiled from 2011 data. Los Angeles, CA: Inter-Agency on Child Abuse and Neglect

cases—less than 8%—in this one county are dismissed, or defendants are either found not guilty or sentenced to probation only. In the majority of cases, almost 65%, perpetrators of fatal child maltreatment serve between 6 years to life. These criminal justice outcomes are harsher than the outcomes that were reported in the 1990s. Since this information is not widely available from other jurisdictions, it is difficult to know if this reflects a larger trend or if it is just related to this one county. Other jurisdictions may also have similarly harsh penalties but just not report them.

Another concern that also focuses on penalties for cases of fatal child maltreatment addresses whether there is parity in the severity of penalties when a child is killed versus when an adult is killed. Anecdotal evidence and media exposés have suggested that when children are victims of maltreatment-related homicides, perpetrators are sentenced to less severe penalties than when adults are victims of homicides. A recent investigation by the Denver Post in Colorado showed that when perpetrators for child versus adult deaths were convicted of comparable crimes, that perpetrators of child deaths had shorter sentences than perpetrators of adult deaths (Augé & Mitchell, 2012). They reported that over a recent 5-year period for class II felonies, perpetrators of adult deaths were, on average, sentenced to 37 years, compared to 30 years for child deaths. Similarly for class III felonies, perpetrators of adult deaths were sentenced to 19 years, compared to 14 years for child deaths. They found that there were even greater discrepancies for sentences of probation or deferred judgment. The information in this exposé was not subject to statistical significance testing to determine the magnitude of the difference in their findings. Such an analysis would have been required in a social science analysis.[1]

Even though investigative journalism shows a difference in sentencing based on the age of the victim, recent social science research does not. Hewes and colleagues (Hewes, Keenan, McDonnell, Dudley, & Herman, 2011) conducted the most comprehensive comparative analysis of criminal justice convictions based on the age of homicide victims. These authors examined criminal justice penalties based on whether homicide victims were children or adults. They analyzed non-law enforcement-related homicides in the state of Utah from 2002 to 2007 and compared 30 child abuse homicide convictions with 112 adult homicide convictions. The research showed conviction rates were similar for child and adult homicides (88.2% and 82%, respectively). Similarly, when criminal justice outcomes were analyzed, while controlling for victim and perpetrator demographic characteristics, there was no difference in the rate of sentencing between cases involving child abuse homicides and adult homicides. This study shows that when cases are brought to trial and when gender or race of the victim and perpetrator are controlled, that there is no difference in sentencing outcomes.

There are some limitations of this study that do not address a number of concerns that are part of the debate on criminal justice outcomes regarding fatal maltreatment. First, because of the nature of the Utah child abuse homicide statute, this study only addresses child *abuse* fatalities and not *neglect* fatalities. Deaths caused by child abuse, as opposed to neglect, usually involve cases that are more violent and perhaps easier to convict by a jury. Second, this study only examined instances where charges were brought against a perpetrator. Previous research has shown that charges are frequently not brought against perpetrators of fatal child maltreatment, especially in cases of neglect (Collins, 2006; Hicks & Gaughan, 1995). Thus, the authors may have a sample of cases where the evidence was especially clear and compelling and this could explain why no differences were found in sentencing between cases involving child death victims and adult death victims. Third, the authors reported that there were differences in sentencing rates before the demographic factors of victims and perpetrators were considered, but those differences and how they might have varied by demographic factors is not reported. This could be important information. Historically, women have received less severe penalties, especially if the child victims were very young (Maier-Katkin & Ogle, 1997; Oberman, 1996; Shelton, Muirhead, & Canning, 2010). Thus, reporting on conviction and sentencing rates by gender and other demographic information would provide useful information to help the field better understand biases that may be at work within the criminal justice system in the conviction and sentencing of perpetrators of fatal child maltreatment.

---

[1] The article did not provide sufficient information for one to conduct these statistical tests of significance.

7.4 The Bottom Line

7.4.1 What We Know

There have been many changes in the criminal justice response to fatal maltreatment in the past several dates. It is unclear how these changes may have an impact on outcomes, but the following is true or is worthy of speculation.

- Despite the many changes in the criminal investigation of children's deaths, these changes are minimally addressed in the professional literature, but the anecdotal evidence of those changes is substantial. Chapter 2 touched on how changes in investigation may be responsible, or in part responsible, for the upward tick in the prevalence rate of fatal child maltreatment. Chapter 9 addresses this further.
- Nevertheless, conflicting approaches to ruling or determining how a child has died remain, which results in unstandardized approaches across the county, individual states, and even counties and other jurisdictions.
- There have been multiple, state-level changes in laws which permit law enforcement professionals to pursue charges of increasingly more serious crimes and that come with harsher penalties in cases of fatal abuse and neglect. This has specifically been true of cases of religiously-motivated medical neglect.

7.4.2 What Remains Unknown

There is very little that we know with certainty about the criminal justice approach and response to fatal child maltreatment. The different approaches to investigating and determining causes of child deaths is anecdotally understood and is increasingly documented in the professional literature, but the extent of these differences and how they have an impact on criminal justice outcomes is unknown.

The changes in child homicide statutes and other portions of the criminal code that allow for harsher charges and penalties to be pursued have not been adequately addressed. We do not know if the changes in these laws have been implemented and if so, if they have resulted in harsher penalties. This is evident through the mixed results regarding whether perpetrators of child homicide versus adult homicide are given similar or different penalties. This issue has rarely been studied and the research that has been conducted has not adequately answered this question. It is important to have this conversation driven by evidence, as opposed to emotion.

In large measure, the literature is silent on whether the changes made within the criminal justice system over the past two to three decades have been effective: how the knowledge and skills of investigators may have changed, if deceased children are better and more accurately identified as victims of maltreatment, if this has resulted in changes in how cases of surviving siblings are handled, and if there have been substantive changes in criminal justice outcomes in cases of fatal child maltreatment. As noted in previous chapters, without evaluation, it is impossible to know whether these efforts have resulted in positive changes regarding the fatal maltreatment of children in the U.S. criminal justice system. This is an area that is ripe for consolidated and consistent practices and approaches, not to mention assessment, evaluation, and research. Without a doubt, there cannot be consensus on these issues without a multipronged approach and cooperation between professional associations, state agencies, experts on the ground, and in academia.

References

American Academy of Pediatrics. (1988). Religious exemptions from child abuse statutes. *Pediatrics, 81*(1), 169–171.
American Academy of Pediatrics. (1997). Religious objections to medical care. *Pediatrics, 99*, 279–281.
American Prosecutors Research Institute. (1994). *Special procedures in child homicide investigations: Mandatory autopsies & child death review teams United States.*
Asser, S., & Swan, R. (1998). Child fatalities from religion motivated medical neglect. *Pediatrics, 101*, 625–629.
Augé, K., & Mitchell, K. (2012, November 16). Short on justice: Penalties for child deaths less severe than for adults in Colorado. *The Denver Post*. Retrieved from http://www.denverpost.com/failedtodeath/ci_21996958/inequity-exists-length-sentences-deaths-kids-and-adults
Bartick, M. (2014, December 19). Pediatric politics: How dire warnings against infant bed sharing "backfired". *WBUR*: Boston's NPR News Station. Retrieved from http://commonhealth.wbur.org/2014/12/dire-warnings-against-infant-bed-sharing-backfired
Bendetowies, B. (1990). Felony murder and child abuse: A proposal for the New York legislature. *Fordham Urban Law Journal, 18*, 383–406.
Biema, D. V. (1998, August 31). Faith or healing? *Time*.
Causey, J. E. (2012, March 10). Should impaired co-sleeping be criminal? *Journal Sentinel*. Retrieved from http://www.jsonline.com/news/opinion/should-impaired-cosleeping-be-criminal-ss4ejn1-142147193.html
Child Abuse Prevention and Treatment Act. (1996), 42 USC 5101; 42 USC 5116, Pub. L. No. 104-235
Children's Healthcare Is a Legal Duty. (2014). *Support HO458: Protect Idaho children from medical neglect*. Retrieved July 30, 2014, from http://childrenshealthcare.org/?page_id=1869
Children's Healthcare Is a Legal Duty. (n.d.-a). *CHILD's public policy achievements*. Retrieved July 31, 2014, from http://childrenshealthcare.org/?page_id=24-Public
Children's Healthcare Is a Legal Duty. (n.d.-b). *Religious exemptions from health care for children*. Retrieved July 31, 2014, from http://childrenshealthcare.org/?page_id=24
Clark, In re: (Common Pleas Court, Lucas County, Ohio 1962).
Collins, J. M. (2006). Crime and parenthood: The uneasy case for prosecuting negligent parents. *Northwestern University Law Review, 100*(2), 807–856.
Commonwealth of Virginia Department for Children. (1990). *Criminal sanctions for child abuse fatalities*. Richmond, VA. Retrieved from http://search.ebscohost.com/login.aspx?direct=true&db=sih&AN=SM126802&site=ehost-live
Cross, T. P., Walsh, W. A., Simone, M., & Jones, L. M. (2003). Prosecution of child abuse: A meta-analysis of rates of criminal justice decisions. *Trauma, Violence & Abuse, 4*(4), 323–340. doi:10.1177/1524838003256561.
Crume, T. L., DiGuiseppi, C., Byers, T., Sirotnak, A. P., & Garrett, C. J. (2002). Underascertainment of child maltreatment fatalities by death certificates, 1990–1998. *Pediatrics, 110*(2), e18.

D'Andrade, A., & Berrick, J. D. (2006). When policy meets practice: The untested effects of permanency reforms in child welfare. *Journal of Sociology and Social Welfare, 33*(1), 31–52.

Dallas Police Department. (1994, August 31–September 2). Paper presented at the crimes against children 1994: The 6th annual seminar presented by the Dallas Police Department & the Dallas Children's Advocacy Center, Dallas, TX.

Davis, S., & Polcyn, B. (2014, July 6). Lawmaker wants blood from parents involved in co-sleeping deaths. *Fox-6-NOW*. Retrieved from http://fox6now.com/2014/07/06/lawmaker-wants-to-hold-drunk-parents-accountable-for-co-sleeping-deaths/

Douglas, E. M. (1999). *The prosecution of fatal child abuse*. Unpublished Manuscript. Portland, ME: Maine Child Abuse Action Network.

Douglas, E. M. (2006). *Mending broken families: Social policies for families of divorce–Are they working?* Lanham, MD: Rowman & Littlefield.

Emery, J. L. (1993). Child abuse, sudden infant death syndrome, and unexpected infant death. *American Journal of Diseases of Children, 147*(10), 1097–1100. doi:10.1001/archpedi.1993.02160340083019.

Ewigman, B., Kivlahan, C., & Land, G. (1993). The Missouri fatality study: Underreporting of maltreatment fatalities among children younger than five years of age, 1983 through 1986. *Pediatrics, 91*(2), 330.

Garstang, J., & Sidebotham, P. (2008). Interagency training: Establishing a course in the management of unexpected childhood death. *Child Abuse Review, 17*(5), 352–361.

Gessner, B. D., Moore, M., Hamilton, B., & Muth, P. T. (2004). The incidence of infant physical abuse in Alaska. *Child Abuse & Neglect, 28*(1), 9–23.

Griffin, L. (2004). "Which one of you did it?" Criminal liability for "causing or allowing" the death of a child. *Indiana International Comparative Law Review, 15*(1), 89–114.

Hamilton, M. (2003). *Why the U.S.'s international religious freedom commission is harming its status in the world community*. Retrieved January 30, 2003, from http://writ.news.findlaw.com/hamilton/20030130.html

Hanzlick, R. L., Jentzen, J. M., & Clark, S. C. (2007). *Sudden, unexplained infant death investigations: Guidelines for the scene investigator*. Atlanta, GA: Centers for Disease Control and Prevention.

Hartog, M. A., Freeman, M., Kubilis, P. S., & Janowski, R. A. (1999). Pediatricians' and social workers' knowledge of Florida's religious immunity laws. *Southern Medical Journal, 92*(4), 632–638.

Herman-Giddens, M. E., Brown, G., Verbiest, S., Carlson, P. J., Hooten, E. G., Howell, E., et al. (1999). Underascertainment of child abuse mortality in the United States. *JAMA, 282*(5), 463–467.

Hewes, H. A., Keenan, H. T., McDonnell, W. M., Dudley, N. C., & Herman, B. E. (2011). Judicial outcomes of child abuse homicide. *Archives of Pediatrics & Adolescent Medicine, 165*(10), 918–921. doi:10.1001/archpediatrics.2011.151.

Hicks, R. A., & Gaughan, D. C. (1995). Understanding fatal child abuse. *Child Abuse & Neglect, 7*, 855–863.

Holmgren, B. K. (2001). Chapter fifteen: Prosecuting the Shaken infant case. *Journal of Aggression, Maltreatment & Trauma, 5*(1), 275–339. doi:10.1300/J146v05n01_15.

Hughes, R. (2014, July 15). Police: Frustrated with his crying, Reading mom kills her baby. *WFMZ-TV69*. Retrieved from http://www.wfmz.com/news/news-regional-berks/police-frustrated-with-his-crying-reading-mom-kills-her-baby/26960656

Huyer, R. (2014, January 21). [Personal communication].

Illinois Dept of Children and Family Services. (1986). *Protocol for child death autopsies*. United States.

Inter-Agency on Child Abuse and Neglect. (2012). *Child death review team report 2012: Report compiled from 2011 data*. Los Angeles, CA: Inter-Agency on Child Abuse and Neglect.

Kaplan, S. R., & Granik, L. A. (1991). *Child fatality investigative procedures manual*. Chicago, IL: American Bar Association.

References

Kim, S. Y., Shapiro-Mendoza, C. K., Chu, S. Y., Camperlengo, L. T., & Anderson, R. N. (2012). Differentiating cause-of-death terminology for deaths coded as sudden infant death syndrome, accidental suffocation, and unknown cause: an investigation using US death certificates, 2003–2004. *Journal of Forensic Sciences, 57*(2), 364–369. doi:10.1111/j.1556-4029.2011.01937.x.

Klevens, J., & Leeb, R. T. (2010). Child maltreatment fatalities in children under 5: Findings from the National Violence Death Reporting System. *Child Abuse & Neglect: The International Journal, 34*(4), 262–266.

Lamparello, A. (2001). Taking god out of the hospital: Requiring parents to seek medical care for their children regardless of religious belief. *Texas Forum on Civil Liberties & Civil Rights, 6*(1), 47–115.

Levene, S., & Bacon, C. J. (2004). Sudden unexpected death and covert homicide in infancy. *Archives of Disease in Childhood, 89*(5), 443–447.

Maier-Katkin, D., & Ogle, R. S. (1997). Policy and disparity: The punishment of infanticide in Britain and America. *International Journal of Comparative & Applied Criminal Justice, 21*(2 special issue), 305–316.

Margolick, D. (1990, August 6). In child deaths, a test for Christian Science. *The New York Times*, p. 1

Mazzola, F., Mohiddin, A., Ward, M., & Holdsworth, G. (2013). How useful are child death reviews: A local area's perspective. *BMC Research Notes, 6*(1), 295–295.

Mills, S., & Kiernan, L. (1998, November 15). Getting away with murder: Many of the child-killers of 1993 are back on the street. *Chicago Tribune*. Retrieved from http://articles.chicagotribune.com/1998-11-15/news/9811180197_1_criminal-justice-system-killers-child

National Center for the Prosecution of Child Abuse. (2013). *Child abuse crimes: Child homicide*. Retrieved December 31, 2014, from http://www.ndaa.org/pdf/ChildHomicide 2013.pdf

National Center for the Review and Prevention of Child Deaths. (n.d.). *CDR reporting*. Retrieved March 28, 2014, from http://www.childdeathreview.org/reporting.htm

North Carolina Child Advocacy Institute. (2005). *Facing the facts: Criminal consequences of child abuse homicide*. Albany, NY: North Carolina Child Advocacy Institute.

Oberman, M. (1996). Mothers who kill: Coming to terms with modern American infanticide. *American Criminal Law Review, 34*, 1.

Parry, R. (2014, June 24). Exclusive: As 11,000 sign petition to release father charged with murder of toddler son who died in 91F car, we reveal the disturbing behavior that will make his supporters think twice. *Mail Online*. Retrieved from http://www.dailymail.co.uk/news/article-2668408/EXCLUSIVE-11-000-signed-petition-release-father-charged-murder-charge-toddler-son-died-91F-car-Here-witnesses-reveal-disturbing-behavior-awful-day-make-supporters-think-twice.html

Phipps, C. A. (1999). Responding to child homicide: A statutory proposal. *The Journal of Criminal Law & Criminology, 89*(2), 535–613.

Prince v. Massachusetts (United States Supreme Court 1944).

Rainey, R. H., & Greer, D. C. (1994). Prosecuting child fatality cases. *The APSAC Advisor, 7*, 28–30.

Rollins, P. A., & Nickerson, G. A. (1978). Prosecuting the child abuse homicide. *Prosecutor, 13*(5), 345–348.

San Diego County Office of the District Attorney. (1977). *Child abuse – A medical/legal training program*. United States.

Sanchez, L., Nock, S. L., Wright, J. D., Pardee, J. W., & Ionescu, M. (2001). The implementation of covenant marriage in Louisiana. *Virginia Journal of Social Policy & Law, 9*(Fall), 192–222.

Scolnick, A. (1990). Religious exemptions to child neglect laws still being passed despite convictions of parents. *JAMA, 264*(10), 1226–1228.

Shapiro-Mendoza, C. K., Camperlengo, L. T., Kim, S. Y., & Covington, T. (2012). The sudden unexpected infant death case registry: A method to improve surveillance. *Pediatrics, 129*(2), 486–493. doi:10.1542/peds.2011-0854.

Shelton, J. L., Muirhead, Y., & Canning, K. E. (2010). Ambivalence toward mothers who kill: An examination of 45 U.S. cases of maternal neonaticide. *Behavioral Sciences & the Law, 28*(6), 812–831. doi:10.1002/bsl.937.

Sirotnak, A. P., & Brittain, C. R. (2006). *Child abuse fatalities understanding the medical diagnosis of child maltreatment: A guide for nonmedical professionals* (3rd ed., pp. 207–213). New York, NY: Oxford University Press.

Soerdjbalie-Maikoe, V., Bilo, R. A. C., van den Akker, E., & Maes, A. (2010). Unnatural death due to child abuse–Forensic autopsies 1996–2009. *Nederlands Tijdschrift Voor Geneeskunde, 154*, A2285–A2285.

Staley, J. (2014, February 13). Baby Brianna ceremonies planned; child's mother could be released in 2016. *Las Cruces Sun News*. Retrieved from http://www.lcsun-news.com/las_cruces-news/ci_25134384/baby-brianna-ceremonies-planned-childs-mother-could-be

Stanton, J., & Simpson, A. (2001). Murder misdiagnosed as SIDS: A perpetrator's perspective. *Archives of Disease in Childhood, 85*(6), 454–459. doi:10.1136/adc.85.6.454.

Stauth, C. (2013). *In the name of God: The true story of the fight to save children from faith-healing homicide*. New York, NY: Thomas Dunne Books/St. Martin's Press.

Stewart, A. M. (1990). Murder by child abuse. *Willamette Law Review, 28*, 435–447.

Swan, R. (1997). Children, medicine, religion and the law. *Advances in Pediatrics, 44*, 491–543.

Swan, R. (1998). On statutes depriving a class of children rights to medical care: Can this discrimination be litigated? *Quinnipiac Health Law, 2*(1), 73–95.

Swan, R. (2010, November). CAPTA reauthorized; almost no improvement on CHILD's issues. *Children's Healthcare Is a Legal Duty, 4*, 1–2.

Tilkin, D. (2013, November 7). Fallen followers: Investigation finds 10 mire dead children of faith healers. *KATU-TV*. Retrieved from http://www.katu.com/news/investigators/Fallen-followers-Investigation-finds-10-more-dead-children-of-faith-healers-231050911.html

U. S. Department of Justice. (2000). *Investigating fatal child abuse & neglect*. United States

United States Advisory Board on Child Abuse and Neglect. (1995). *A nation's shame: Fatal child abuse and neglect in the United States*.

Vollrath, D. R. (2011). Shaken baby syndrome as felony murder in North Carolina. *Campbell Law Review, 34*, 423.

Walsh, B. (2005). *Investigating child fatalities. Portable guides in investigating child abuse*. Washington, DC: Office of Juvenile Justice and Delinquency Prevention.

Washoe County Child Death Review Team. (n.d.). *Agency roles for investigating suspicious child deaths and serious injuries*. Washoe County, NV: Washoe County Child Death Review Team.

Westveer, A. E. (1997). *Managing death investigation*. Washington, DC: U. S. Federal Bureau of Investigation.

Chapter 8
Prevention of Fatal Child Maltreatment: What Are We Doing That Is Working?

The final policy, programmatic, and professional response that this book addresses is prevention. Most efforts in this arena have concerned the prevention of child abuse or neglect in general, because if one prevents the maltreatment of children then obviously, abuse or neglect-related deaths are also prevented. There have also been some efforts to educate parents or the general public about certain types of caregiving behaviors that might especially place a child at-risk for fatality, such as shaking a baby or leaving a child unattended in a vehicle. These programs and their effectiveness will be the focus of this chapter. Throughout this book, I have started each chapter by outlining the areas of controversy or disagreement in the field. Contention or disagreement, especially as it relates to fatal child maltreatment, are not present in the area of child maltreatment prevention.

8.1 Levels of Prevention

As noted in Chapter 1, the field of public health defines prevention on three levels (Centers for Disease Control & Prevention, n.d.; Starfield, Hyde, Gérvas, & Heath, 2008). Briefly, primary prevention focuses on preventing the onset of a disease or a condition among the general population. Secondary prevention focuses on prevention among those who are at-risk for a condition or who are experiencing early symptoms of a condition or a disease. Tertiary prevention focuses on minimizing consequences of, arresting, or preventing the reoccurrence of a condition or disease. This model is often a point of reference in discussions of prevention programs.

8.2 Previous Recommendations to Prevent Maltreatment Fatalities

Two previous books have addressed the prevention of fatal child maltreatment: Cyril Greenland's (1989) *Preventing CAN Deaths: An International Study of Deaths Due to Child Abuse and Neglect* and Sharon Vincent's (2010b) *Preventing Child Deaths: Learning from Review*. Both of these books, penned years apart, offer recommendations for change and ways to potentially prevent fatal child maltreatment. Greenland's book was published when western nations were just beginning to turn their attention to issues concerning death by abuse and neglect and his work was part of the increasing call for new approaches to prevent maltreatment fatalities. Trained as a clinical social worker, his attention was often focused on individual characteristics or treatments for children or parents. At the same time, it was likely his own professional experience in the deinstitutionalization of psychiatric hospitals in Canada that allowed him to recognize the importance of larger systems issues in the prevention of child maltreatment fatalities (CMFs). More than 25 years ago he noted the importance of child welfare workers collaborating with professionals outside of their agencies and reinforced the hugely significant role that multidisciplinary teams could, and have come to play in the context of addressing abuse and neglect at the societal level. His recommendations largely focused on secondary and tertiary prevention—preventing deaths among at-risk families or in families where children are already experiencing abuse or neglect—both of which are addressed in this chapter.

Vincent's recommendations, which are the result of a two-part series of books (Vincent, 2010a, 2010b) exclusively focused on the unique role that child death review plays in the investigation of unexplained children's deaths in the United Kingdom, Australia, New Zealand, the United States, and Canada (see Chapter 5 for more information). Her recommendations focus on large-scale reforms within the public child protection systems in these countries and changes that have occurred within their respective legislative bodies. That said, her final words include recommendations for the adoption of a broad primary prevention for all children, such as home visiting programs, which are reviewed later in this chapter.

8.3 State and County Programs

A number of states have launched initiatives to reduce the incidence of child deaths in their respective states. Alabama and North Carolina have both taken this approach through different means, but appear to have had successful outcomes. Alabama, which attributes its decline in child deaths to their state's child death review team, has seen a decline in deaths, specifically among older children in vehicular accidents and infants who die from "positional sleep issues" (Oliver, 2014). They have seen declines in the raw number of children who have died, but did not present information about the rate at which children die. Deaths due to positional sleep issues are likely related to CMFs as a potential form of neglect, but again, without documenting the rate of these deaths one cannot conclude that change has been made. North Carolina established the Child Fatality Task Force as a legislative study commission; their child fatality rate has been cut in half between 1990 and 2012 (North Carolina Child Fatality Task Force, 2014b). It is unclear how CMFs are presented in this data, but a brief slice of data from 2008 to 2012 shows an increase in homicide among children (North Carolina Child Fatality Task Force, 2014a).

The Sacramento County Child Death Review Team (2012) conducted a 20 year analysis of child death data from 1990 to 2010, in which they link CMF deaths directly to prevention programs: "Child Abuse and Neglect (CAN) homicides fluctuate in direct relationship to funding for programs to prevent them. When services are available, CAN Homicides [sic] decline. When services are cut or reduced, CAN Homicides [sic] increase" (p. ix). In this scenario, the authors argued that when funding for parent education or early home visiting services is present, the raw number of CMFs in Sacramento County decreased and when this funding was withdrawn, the raw number of CMFs increased. The authors of the report acknowledge that conducting research without the proper controls to establish this relationship is beyond the scope of the review team's activities, but they further state "[T]he conclusion that effective programs do make a difference is bolstered by the demonstrated impact of other programs in Sacramento County such as car seat safety, shaken baby syndrome, and infant safe sleeping education programs that, when funded, have also resulted in significant reductions in child deaths" (p. ix). At this time, there is insufficient evidence to conclude that social service programming in Sacramento County could be linked to actual declines in the rate of CMFs.

8.4 Prevention Programs That Are Specific to Fatal Child Maltreatment

This section of the chapter addresses techniques that have been used to specifically address the death or serious injury of children. These are programs that largely deal with primary prevention at the individual level or through large, public education campaigns. Research that I conducted with a colleague on the recommendations that emerged from child death review teams showed a high level of concern regarding the need for more public education about the safety of children in a variety of settings (Douglas & Cunningham, 2008). The two areas that received the most attention concerned shaken baby syndrome (SBS) (or abusive head trauma—AHT) and water safety.

8.4.1 Shaken Baby Syndrome/Abusive Head Trauma

The leading prevention and education campaigns that most specifically address fatalities and that most directly result from increased attention to fatal child maltreatment are those that address traumatic brain injury or what is commonly called

SBS/AHT (Douglas, 2005). Both the Centers for Disease Control & Prevention and the American Academy of Pediatrics identify SBS as a form of traumatic brain injury (American Academy of Pediatrics, 2009; Centers for Disease Control & Prevention, 2012); it is described as a severe form of physical child abuse in which an infant is violently shaken by the arms, legs, chest, or shoulders. Infants essentially suffer from an inflicted whiplash injury, that results in bleeding inside the brain and behind the eyes (Carbaugh, 2004). Injuries can also be inflicted by blunt trauma to the head, hence, the American Academy of Pediatrics' recommendation for the use of the broader term, "abusive head trauma" (American Academy of Pediatrics, 2009).

This violent act has been the target of repeated primary prevention campaign efforts throughout the country: through media—including television broadcasting, posters, and pamphlets, and has been supported by politicians, government agencies, nonprofit organizations, professionals, and victims' families. This widespread support has been demonstrated in New York City with the support of then-mayor Michael Bloomberg (New York City Administration for Children's Services, 2002) and in Alabama, where the state's child death review team sponsors a SBS awareness campaign (Durfee, Durfee, & West, 2002). The National Exchange Club distributes brochures, billboards, magnets and T-shirts about preventing abusive head trauma, as part of their child maltreatment public awareness campaigns (see http://www.preventchildabuse.com/). The organization, "Don't Shake Jake," was founded and is run by a Maine family whose infant son, Jake, died from SBS, perpetrated by his babysitter (see http://www.dontshakejake.org/).

Hospital-based primary prevention programs for SBS/AHT have been conducted at increasing levels since the turn of the twenty-first century. A growing body of research has emerged since this time, which provides promising support for the efficacy of hospital-based primary prevention of SBS and/or AHT. The first scholar to show evidence of the effectiveness of this work was completed by Mark Dias and colleagues (Dias et al., 2005). The seminal piece of work focused on hospital-based, primary prevention in eight counties in western New York State. Parents of newborns were provided information about the dangers of shaking an infant and alternatives to shaking when a baby persistently cries. The parents were asked to sign a commitment letter indicating that they had received this information and that they understood it. In addition, the hospital placed posters in the building about the dangers of shaking a baby. Seven months post-education, the vast majority of parents remembered that shaking an infant was harmful. Further, the authors compared the rate of SBS 6 years before intervention (1993–1998), with 5 years post-intervention (1999–2003), and found a 47% reduction in the incidence of SBS per 100,000 live births. These results were compared with several counties in neighboring Pennsylvania, which did not implement the SBS/AHT education program. These counties had no decline in the incidence of SBS.

Research since this time has examined many other aspects of SBS prevention programs (Barr, 2012): the process by which hospitals and other organizations implement a primary prevention program to reduce the incidence of SBS (Smith & deGuehery, 2008), what method of delivery is most effective (reading material,

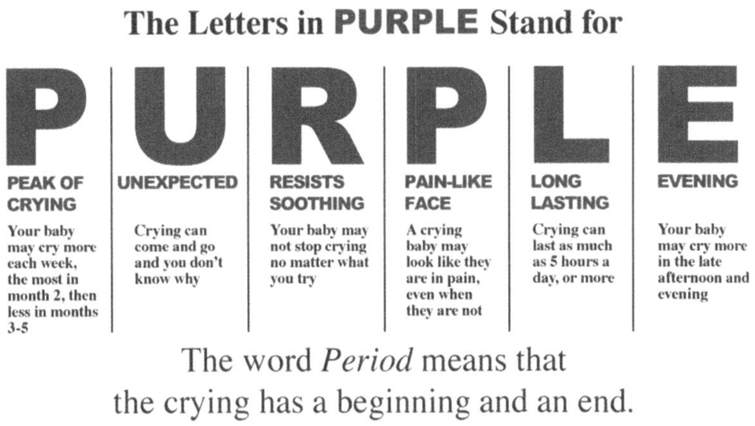

The Letters in **PURPLE** Stand for

P|U|R|P|L|E

PEAK OF CRYING	**UNEXPECTED**	**RESISTS SOOTHING**	**PAIN-LIKE FACE**	**LONG LASTING**	**EVENING**
Your baby may cry more each week, the most in month 2, then less in months 3-5	Crying can come and go and you don't know why	Your baby may not stop crying no matter what you try	A crying baby may look like they are in pain, even when they are not	Crying can last as much as 5 hours a day, or more	Your baby may cry more in the late afternoon and evening

The word *Period* means that the crying has a beginning and an end.

Figure 8.1 The *Period of Purple Crying*, National Center on Shaken Baby Syndrome

video, etc.) (Russell, Trudeau, & Britner, 2008), how well parents retain this information, and whether parents and hospital staff respond positively to the prevention program (Reese, Heiden, Kim, & Yang, 2014). Additionally, studies have continued to confirm that these prevention programs are associated with declines in the prevalence of SBS (Altman et al., 2011).

A more recent contribution to this approach has been to incorporate more information on the crying behaviors of young infants. The *PURPLE* program refers to a phenomenon which has been termed the "*Period of PURPLE Crying*," which describes the period from about 2 weeks of age to 4–5 months when babies often cry the most (Barr, Barr et al., 2009; Barr, Rivara et al., 2009; Runyan et al., 2009). As Figure 8.1 shows, the acronym *PURPLE* stands for: P=Peak of crying, U=Unexpected, R=Resists soothing, P=Pain-like face, L=Long-lasting, and E=evening time. In addition to educating parents about the harmful effects of shaking an infant and the alternatives to shaking, this primary prevention program emphasizes that infants often cry for no apparent reason. The curriculum educates parents that infant crying occurs as part of a normal developmental stage and does not imply that infants are sick or that parents are ineffective. Instead, it reframes the issue of early infant crying as something that can be expected and helps to prepare parents for this stage and the possible frustrations that go with it. The *PURPLE* program has also been highlighted by the Centers for Disease Control & Prevention (Centers for Disease Control & Prevention, n.d.).

As I have written before (Douglas, 2005), it is not well documented why SBS has become the leading prevention campaign that has emerged from the increased awareness on fatal child maltreatment. It may be because SBS/AHT affects the most vulnerable children and because health and service providers have fairly easy access to families with young infants, right after childbirth. Moreover, SBS can result from one-time incidents of rage, as opposed to chronic maltreatment; thus, parents may be more receptive to learning about this form of maltreatment and strategies for prevention. Finally, more than 50% of SBS/AHT cases are perpetrated by nonparental caregivers (Starling & Holden, 1995)—another piece of information that may convince parents about the importance of learning about this phenomenon. In short, the success of SBS prevention programs may be strongly related to access to potential victims and the receptiveness of parents to learn prevention techniques.

Indeed, parents are open to and rarely resist learning about SBS; they report finding it helpful, and their retention of the information is encouraging (Barr, Barr, et al., 2009; Reese et al., 2014; Shanahan et al., 2014; Stoll & Anderson, 2013). Nurses are also open to incorporating SBS/AHT information into their work routines and interactions with parents of new infants (Stewart et al., 2011; Stoll & Anderson, 2013). Research shows that using a multi-prong approach to educate families is most effective—with direct education to nursing staff and parents and large-scale public education (Barr, 2012; Runyan et al., 2009; Stewart et al., 2011); additionally, parents learn about SBS most effectively when information is provided through video, as opposed to written material only (Russell et al., 2008). The most important outcome is that research shows that instances of SBS decline when prevention programs are put in place (Altman et al., 2011; Dias et al., 2005).

Seventeen states have passed legislation mandating, encouraging, or permitting information about SBS/AHT in hospitals or birthing centers in their states. Additionally, 12 states have provisions concerning public education about the prevention of SBS (National Conference of State Legislatures, 2014), an example of which is shown in Figure 8.2. Several areas of SBS/AHT prevention programs could benefit from revision or program improvement. Nurses do not always emphasize that infant crying peaks around 2 months (Shanahan et al., 2014); additionally, there are mixed findings regarding whether parents share the information that they have learned about SBS with other caregivers of their children (Barr, Barr, et al., 2009; Shanahan et al., 2014), which is important because of the high proportion of non-family caregivers who perpetrate SBS/AHT. Finally, given the high success rate of SBS prevention programs, it warrants being mandated in every state by statute.

8.4.2 Supervision of Children

As noted throughout this book, most children who die from maltreatment, die from neglect, as opposed to abuse. Yet, with the exception of primary prevention public service announcements about water safety and leaving children in cars alone, there has been little effort to educate the public concerning the need to supervise children. Water safety has probably been given the most attention, as evidenced by some literature which assesses parents' knowledge about water safety (Lee & Thompson, 2007; Morrongiello, Sandomierski, & Spence, 2014; Simon, Tamura, & Colton, 2003). This small body of literature shows that some parents leave small children unattended, for brief periods of time, while they are bathing. Between 5 and 15% of

8.4 Prevention Programs That Are Specific to Fatal Child Maltreatment

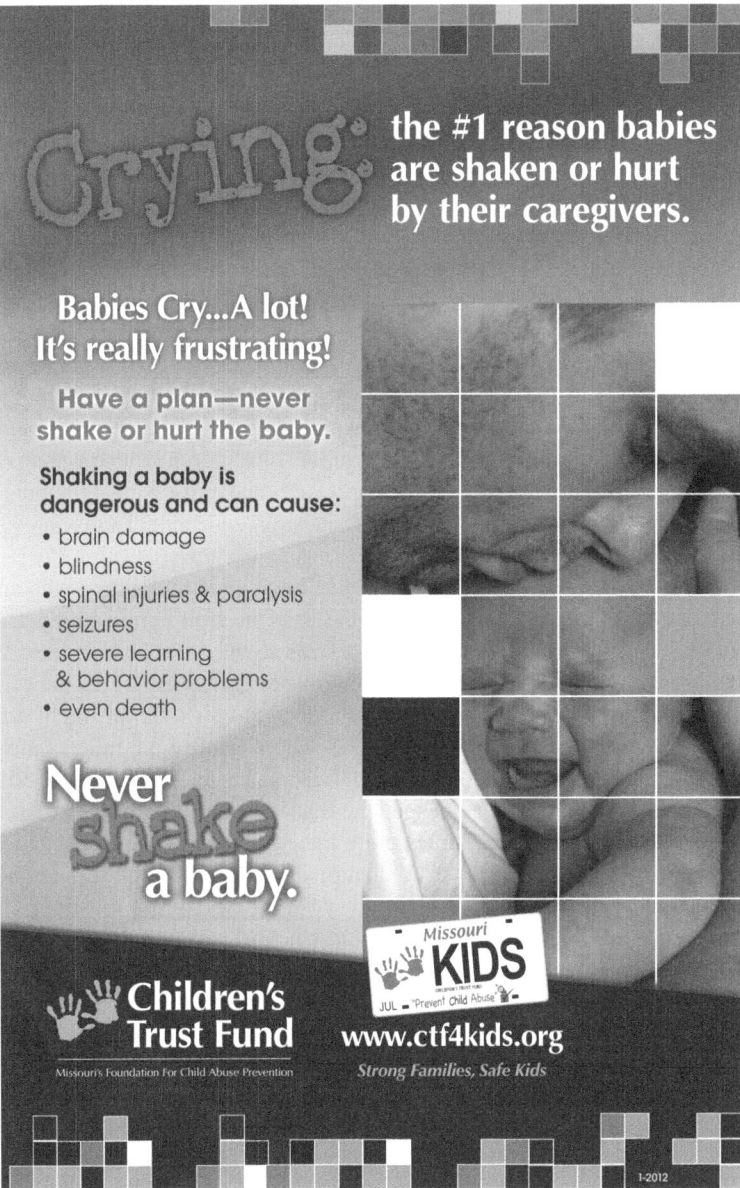

Figure 8.2 Example of Shaken Baby Syndrome Public Education Prevention Initiative, Missouri Children's Trust Fund

parents of infants reported leaving their children unattended while bathing while they attended to a household task (Lee & Thompson, 2007; Simon et al., 2003); this was true for up to one-third of parents of children under the age of 5 (Simon et al., 2003).

Parents' willingness to leave their children unsupervised around water may be due to a lack of education in this area. A study of over 300 pediatric and family health professionals found that only one-third counsel parents about risk factors for drowning and the importance of practicing water safety with children (Barkin & Gelberg, 1999). This speaks to the potential importance of educating both professionals and caregivers about drowning prevention. One study found that parents of children ages 2–5 who were engaged in swimming classes, were increasingly, but falsely, confident in their children's ability to protect themselves around water (Morrongiello et al., 2014). They recommended that parent education about water safety be integrated into children's swim lessons. The Drowning Prevention Foundation (http://drowningpreventionfoundation.com/) and the Centers for Disease Control and Prevention (2014c) provide information about water safety and how to avoid drowning, but there is no concentrated, national effort regarding supervising children around water to prevent drowning. Overall, there is very little literature concerning water safety, how failing to supervise children around water is often a form of neglect, the need to educate caregivers and professionals about water safety, and almost no literature on the efficacy of education and/or prevention programs.

As of late, an increasing level of attention is being paid to children who are left in cars unattended. Most of this concerns the extreme heat temperatures that can occur in cars that are left in the sun and children dying from heat stroke (Agran, 1991; Guard & Gallagher, 2005; McLaren, Null, & Quinn, 2005). Some of these cases have resulted in the criminal prosecution of parents who left their children unattended (Armagost, 2001; Collins, 2006). The organization called Safe Kids Worldwide (2014) reports that 23% of parents report having left children under the age of 4, alone inside parked cars, despite the risks associated with heatstroke. They also report that fathers are three times more likely to leave children unattended in vehicles than mothers. One effort to combat this has been a public education campaign launched by the U.S. National Highway Traffic Safety Administration (n.d.) that promotes the phrase: *"Where's baby? Look before you lock!"* that is displayed in Figure 8.3. Numerous other organizations and states have also launched their own initiatives, including "Kids & Cars" (http://www.kidsandcars.org/) and some of the state-level Children's Trust Funds promote awareness about leaving children in vehicles unattended. The professional literature does not document if parent education or public service announcements have been effective in educating caregivers, changing attitudes, prompting behavior changes on the part of caregivers or bystand-

Figure 8.3 Example of Public Education to Promote Safe Supervision of Children in Cars, U.S. National Highway Traffic Safety Administration

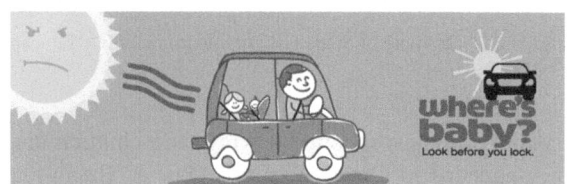

ers, or in reducing the rate of children being left unattended in vehicles or suffering from heatstroke or dying.

There is a small body of literature that addresses inadequate caregiver supervision of children and its relationship to children's injuries and deaths (Damashek, Drass, & Bonner, 2014; Morrongiello, Corbett, McCourt, & Johnston, 2006; Peterson, 1994). But, there is no widespread, national or state primary prevention campaign that addresses the importance of supervising children, or any evaluation of such a campaign, pilot project, or the like. Such efforts may exist somewhere, but if so, they are not well known to professionals in the field.

8.4.3 Safe Sleeping Environments for Children

There has recently been an increased attention to safe sleeping environments for infants. For example, Ohio states that every week, three infants die because of unsafe sleeping environments (Ohio Department of Health, 2014b). The co-sleeping of infants with family members and/or family pets is often linked to fatalities and this has caught the attention of many health professionals (American Academy of Pediatrics, 2011). Further, I know from anecdotal evidence and from the websites of state offices of child and family services (New York State Office of Children and Family Services, 2014) that some child welfare agencies tell parents that it is not safe to co-sleep with their infants. It places their infants at-risk for death. These would be examples of secondary and tertiary prevention when the information targets families working within the child welfare system. Within the past few years, some states, such as Wisconsin, Washington, Ohio, and Nevada have been sponsoring large-scale, primary prevention, public service announcements that warn about the dangers of co-sleeping and instead promote the ABC of safe sleep: *Alone*, on his/her *Back*, and in a *Crib* (Dell'Antonia, 2011; Ohio Department of Health, 2014a; Stephenson, 2011; "This PSA shows why it's best for babies to sleep alone," 2014; Watts, 2013). Figure 8.4 shows Ohio's efforts to combat this problem. To date, there has been no research to document the effectiveness of these efforts.

8.5 Prevention of Child Abuse and Neglect, in General

This book focuses on fatal child maltreatment, and thus, this chapter is primarily concerned with how to prevent fatalities. That said, if we are able to prevent child maltreatment, in general, then, by extension, we would obviously also prevent CMFs. There have been a variety of child maltreatment prevention programs in place for the last half-century or more. The Centers for Disease Control and Prevention (2014a) have recently highlighted some of these programs, which are discussed in more detail in the following pages. Most programs have come in one of two forms: prevention services to children and families and parent education/preparation, both of which are reviewed here with regard to their effectiveness in preventing maltreatment.

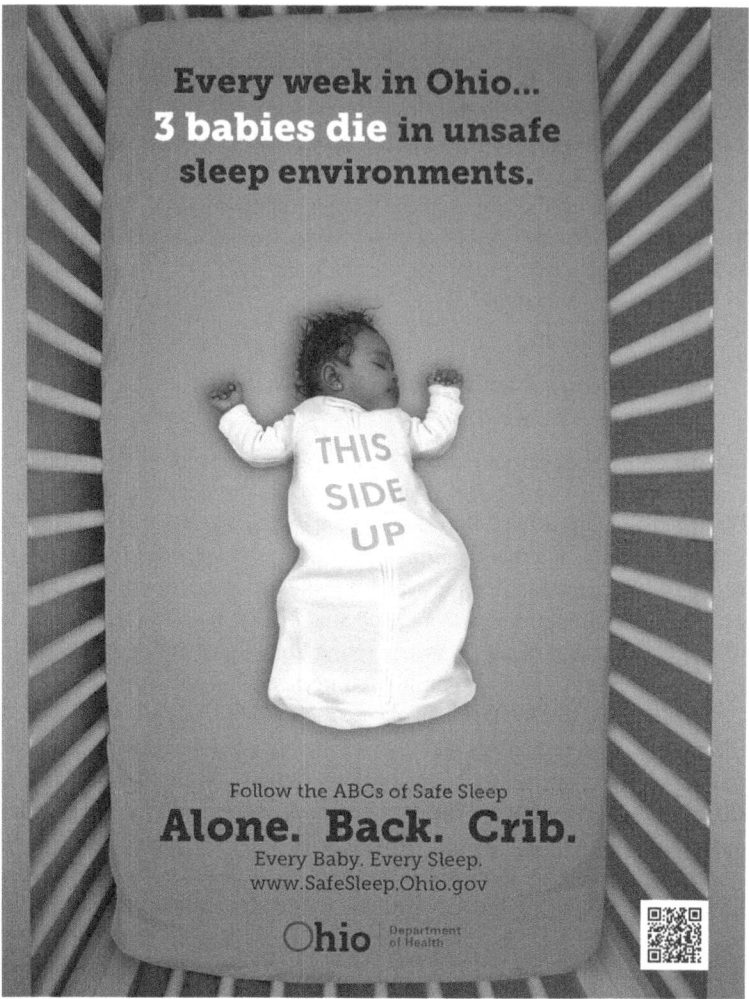

Figure 8.4 Example of the *ABC* of Safe Sleep for Infants Public Education, Ohio Department of Health

8.5.1 Prevention Services

The most common type of prevention services have been offered in families' homes. For example, early home visitation services is a type of program in which parents of new children receive in-home services about child development, parenting, the parent-child relationship, and other information, such as how to receive social welfare services, developing and maintaining healthy relationships, and the like (Guterman, 2001). Home visiting services can be offered by para-professionals, social workers, or nurses. Further, they can be offered as a method of primary prevention, where services are offered to the general public, as was the case in Vermont in the 1990s (Canellos, 2003). Or, they can be a method of secondary prevention, where services are targeted to at-risk families (Bidgood & van de Sande, 1990). The duration over which families are served varies considerably. It can range from a single visit after the birth of a child, to services that start before birth and terminate when the child is about a year old (Bidgood & van de Sande, 1990; Guterman, 2001; Halpern, 1986).

The early literature on home visiting programs was very promising. Research found that parents who received home visiting services were less likely to be the subject of a report made to child protective services (Eckenrode, 2000; Green, Power, Steinbook, & Gaines, 1981; Guterman, 1999; Olds, Henderson, Chamberlin, & Tatelbaum, 1986). Not all research was this favorable, however, (Marcenko & Spence, 1994) and study design varied substantially (Chaffin, 2004). Today, the professional literature largely shows that early home visiting programs have little ability to protect a child from experiencing maltreatment, especially among the highest risk populations, which receive secondary or tertiary prevention services (Filene, Kaminski, Valle, & Cachat, 2013; Goyal, Teeters, & Ammerman, 2013; McFarlane et al., 2010; Sweet & Appelbaum, 2004). Despite these limitations, scholars and practitioners, alike, began to emphasize the connection between home visiting programs and the promotion of more positive parenting techniques, less hazardous living environments, and healthier children—all of which reduce the risk for maltreatment (Guterman, 1999, 2001; MacLeod & Nelson, 2000; Olds, Henderson, & Kitzman, 1994; Olds & Kitzman, 1993).

Today, home visiting programs are receiving significant federal support. The Centers for Disease Control & Prevention have recommended and funded a number of programs as a potential way to prevent child maltreatment (Centers for Disease Control & Prevention, 2014a, 2014b) and a number of state programs are funded through a provision of the Affordable Care Act (U.S. Department of Health & Human Services, 2013). This national home visiting agenda is perhaps best demonstrated by the website called Home Visiting Evidence of Effectiveness (http://homvee.acf.hhs.gov/), which is sponsored by the U.S. Department of Health & Human Services, Administration for Children & Families. This website provides information on hundreds of studies and allows one to search for outcomes in specific areas, such as preventing child maltreatment, maternal health, child health, economic sufficiency, etc. This compilation of information regarding home visiting programs also shows that home visiting programs have not been especially effective in preventing child abuse or neglect. The outliers are: Child FIRST in Connecticut, Nurse-Family Partnership, and SafeCare Augmented, which have all shown fewer substantiation of child abuse or neglect by child welfare agencies.

The Nurse-Family Partnership has been in existence for decades and has been the subject of randomized control studies. In the 21 studies conducted using the Nurse-Family Partnership, one found that at the 15 year follow up, families were less likely to have been substantiated for child abuse and neglect (Olds, Eckenrode, Henderson et al., 1997). There was also a relatively recent publication by Olds and colleagues (Olds et al., 2014) that assessed the efficacy of the Nurse-Family Partnership in preventing child fatalities over a 21-year period of time, after a 2-year home visiting, randomized intervention. Three preventable child fatalities were examined: unintentional injury, sudden infant death syndrome (SIDS), and homicide. The results showed that nine children in the control group died from preventable causes and zero (none) from the intervention group died. The authors caution about drawing strong conclusions because of the small sample size. This is the first study that has linked home visiting services to fatalities, but it is important to remind readers that this study was not specifically about CMFs; even homicides could have been perpetrated by individuals outside the home.

In a randomized control study, families working with the Child FIRST program showed a lower rate of involvement with child protective services 36 months post-baseline involvement (Lowell, Carter, Godoy, Paulicin, & Briggs-Gowan, 2011). This is the only evaluation that is available on this program. Finally, an expanded version of SafeCare, called SafeCare-Augmented was used with families in rural settings. Using random assignment to SafeCare, SafeCare-Augmented, or a control group, those families receiving the augmented version of SafeCare were less likely to have reports to child welfare services concerning children exposed to domestic violence (Silovsky et al., 2011). A handful of other programs have also found a reduction in parent self-report of abusive and neglectful behaviors, but nothing which was independently confirmed by child protective services (Drazen & Haust, 1993; Duggan et al., 2004, 2007; Dumont et al., 2010; Fergusson, Horwood, & Ridder, 2005).

Today, the professional literature largely shows that early home visiting programs show little efficacy in protecting a child from experiencing maltreatment, especially among the highest risk populations (Chaffin, 2004; Filene et al., 2013; Goyal et al., 2013; McFarlane et al., 2010; Sweet & Appelbaum, 2004). That said, there are a number of promising programs and more rigorous and higher quality research is being conducted on these programs. When viewed from a fatal child maltreatment lens, the literature provides limited support to indicate that home visiting programs can currently help reduce the incidence of fatal child maltreatment. Home visiting programs do provide other supports to children and families, so there is no reason to recommend a discontinuation of their use, but helping professionals and decision-makers, alike, would be remiss to believe that these programs provide solid evidence to help prevent fatal child abuse or neglect.

8.5.2 Parenting Education

There have been many, many attempts to prevent the onset or reoccurrence of child maltreatment through some form of parent education or parent intervention. Widely used by child welfare agencies as part of a family's service plan (Gelles, 1996), there has generally been little empirical support for these programs. More recently, such programs have been built on or informed by research and there are several that empirically provide support for the reduction of child maltreatment.

8.5 Prevention of Child Abuse and Neglect, in General

The makers of Positive Parenting Program, or Triple P, market themselves as being able to give parents tools to become the parents that they want to be, with guarantees to help parents raise, happy, healthy, and confident children, to learn to positively manage misbehavior, and to set rules that respects the wishes of everyone in the family—all the while, helping parents take care of themselves and to have confidence in their parenting techniques (Triple P, n.d.-b). Triple P is one of the few programs that has found positive outcomes in parent and child behavior, and that has been found to reduce the likelihood of physical abuse (Poole, Seal, & Taylor, 2014). Triple P, which first appears in the professional literature in 1999, was created by Matt Sanders in Australia. One of the most unique aspects of Triple P is that it offers a suite of programs across different populations, so that prevention is conducted at the primary, secondary, and tertiary levels (Barth, 2009; Triple P, n.d.-c). In fact, the creator of Triple P has argued on many occasions about the importance of using a universal and targeted approach to parenting education in order to promote child and family well-being (Sanders, 2012; Sanders & Kirby, 2014; Sanders & Pidgeon, 2011).

There is a plethora of research that shows the impact of the Triple P program in increasing positive parenting behaviors, increasing parents' self-esteem, decreasing child behavior problems, and parenting stress (Bodenmann, Cina, Ledermann, & Sanders, 2008; Heinrichs, Kliem, & Hahlweg, 2014; Mazzucchelli & Sanders, 2011; Sanders, 1999; Sanders, Kirby, Tellegen, & Day, 2014; Sanders et al., 2004), even in different nations (Bodenmann et al., 2008; de Graaf, Speetjens, Smit, de Wolff, & Tavecchio, 2008).

The effectiveness of Triple P was tested in a population-based trial, where 18 counties in a southeastern US state were randomly assigned to an intervention treatment of Triple P or a control condition—services as usual (Prinz, Sanders, Shapiro, Whitaker, & Lutzker, 2009). In this study, all five levels of Triple P were implemented across the counties, from public service announcements to programs for families at risk of maltreatment; primary, secondary, and tertiary prevention. The counties that focused on providing Triple P to the community experienced 340 fewer cases of substantiated child maltreatment, 240 fewer foster care placements, and 60 fewer injuries caused by child maltreatment injury as determined by hospitals and emergency rooms—as compared with the counties without the intervention (Barth, 2009; Prinz et al., 2009). A recent review of the literature addressed the ability of universal parenting education programs that used a media component, to reduce the potential for physical child abuse (Poole et al., 2014); the authors cautiously endorsed Triple P as a program that holds promise.

At the individual-level, the research on Triple P has been very promising for a number of child and families outcomes (Sanders, Kirby, et al., 2014; Sanders et al., 2004). That said, the research on Triple P's ability to reduce active child maltreatment or to reduce re-reports to child welfare agencies is limited (Barth, 2009; Sanders & Pidgeon, 2011). Further, the research appears to be primarily focused on preventing child physical abuse, as opposed to neglect, which is the primary reason why children die in maltreating families.

Parent-child interaction therapy (PCIT) is a parent training program that provides secondary and tertiary prevention services; it focuses on building and strengthening the parent-child dyad (Funderburk & Elherg, 2011) through observation of parent-child interactions, along with live-feedback for parents during treatment (Urquiza & McNeil, 1996). A number of studies have showed a positive relationship between PCIT and reductions in being at-risk for and in actual child maltreatment (Chaffin, Funderburk, Bard, Valle, & Gurwitch, 2011; Chaffin et al., 2004; Timmer, Urquiza, Zebell, & McGrath, 2005). For example, one study examined 110 parents who had confirmed reports of physical child abuse (Chaffin et al., 2004). These parents were randomly assigned to traditional parenting services in the community or approximately 20 sessions of PCIT. These families were followed for two-and-a-half years after treatment completion; results showed that 19% parents who had received the PCIT condition had re-reports for physical child abuse, compared to 49% of parents in the control group. Other research in PCIT has shown decreases in child abuse potential (Thomas, 2011; Thomas & Zimmer-Gembeck, 2012) and in combination with other intervention methods, such as motivational interviewing, as a way to reduce re-reports of physical child abuse to child welfare agencies (Chaffin et al., 2011).

PCIT and other interventions, such as parent-infant psychotherapy or child-infant psychotherapy (Barnett, Rosenberg, Rosenberg, Osofsky, & Wolford, 2014; Willheim, 2013; Wright, 1986) largely focus on the way that parents interact with their children and this squarely taps into the set of risk factors for CMF that focus on the parent-child relationship (Fein, 1979). This is an area which I have noted before deserves more attention (Douglas, 2005, 2015). Because of the relational part of this treatment, it is more appropriately geared toward abuse than neglect; in fact, PCIT has been shown to have little effect on child welfare reports focusing on neglect (Chaffin et al., 2004), thus, its capacity to address neglect-related fatalities is likely insufficient.

8.6 The Bottom Line

8.6.1 *What We Know*

In the area of fatal child maltreatment prevention, we don't know much. The picture doesn't really improve when we add in the prevention of child maltreatment, in general. But, what we do know is important and could hold wide-ranging implications for the health and safety of children in the United States. There is good evidence that SBS prevention programs work, specifically the program by Mark Dias (2005) and the *PURPLE* Program (Barr, Barr, et al., 2009; Barr, Rivara, et al., 2009; Reese et al., 2014). What is most worrying about this good news is that according to the National Conference of State Legislatures (2014), only 13 states mandate birthing centers to provide SBS prevention education to new parents; 11 states mandate public education about SBS; only eight states require child care providers to be trained in techniques to prevent SBS; and only two states mandate that SBS content be delivered to youth in secondary schools. Given what we know about the effectiveness of these programs to change parent knowledge, parent behavior, and actually prevent cases of SBS, this type of education should be mandated in every state in the Union.

We also know that with regard to preventing non-fatal child physical abuse, Triple P appears to be a promising program (Poole et al., 2014; Prinz et al., 2009; Sanders, Kirby, et al., 2014). Further, the parent training program, PCIT, also appears to reduce the likelihood of reports of physical abuse to child protective agencies, at the secondary and tertiary level—those at-risk for and with confirmed cases of abuse (Chaffin et al., 2004, 2011; Thomas, 2011). Of course, these programs would likely have the potential to also prevent fatal physical abuse as well. The most promising home visiting programs that offer secondary and tertiary prevention services are Child FIRST, Nurse-Family Partnership and an augmented version of SafeCare. Finally, the Nurse-Family Partnership has promising results that it could reduce fatalities, but this is not specific to only CMFs (Olds et al., 2014).

8.6.2 What Remains Unknown

Without a doubt, the flip side of knowing little, is that there remains a lot left to learn. The field in the area of fatal child maltreatment prevention is largely wide-open. At the beginning of this chapter, I highlighted some state initiatives to reduce child deaths. Any states or counties that work to reduce children's fatalities are to be applauded, but often times it is difficult to assess the efficacy of their activities because deaths are often reported in raw numbers and because CMFs are such a rare event. Changes in children's deaths should be reported as both raw numbers and rates, per 100,000 live children because the rate takes into account the changing size of the population. Further, these initiatives do not always report on the different causes of death, making it difficult to determine which prevention efforts may be having the most significant impact. An excellent example of this is the endorsement of the Nurse-Family Partnership by the U.S. Commission to End Child Abuse and Neglect Fatalities. It was heralded as the "only…practice with research evidence showing a reduction in fatalities" (U.S. Commission to End Child Abuse and Neglect Fatalities, 2016, p. 10). While this statement is true, it is not accurate that the Nurse-Family Partnership helps to reduce deaths caused by abuse or neglect, specifically, because this has never been examined.

There is a significant amount of time and attention put into primary prevention public service announcements regarding the importance of supervising children around water, the dangers of leaving children unattended in vehicles, and in having infants co-sleep with family members or pets. But, we have no idea if these measures increase knowledge, change behavior, or reduce the incidence rate of deaths.

Difficult as it might be to examine the long-term effects of such an approach, this is an area ripe for attention from researchers in the field, who could begin with assessing potential changes in knowledge, attitudes, and self-reported behavior.

On a related note, it is probably safe to say that the public and parents alike, think that most children die from abuse, as opposed to neglect. Informing the public about the manner in which most children die may be a first step in working to reduce fatalities. It might promote behavior change and increase vigilance concerning the physical safety of children in their most immediate environments—their homes, vehicles, bathrooms, and sleeping environments.

There is no evidence that any child maltreatment prevention or parenting education program helps to prevent childhood neglect. In the past, the field backed some home visiting programs that were thought to prevent neglect, but there isn't strong enough evidence to endorse this approach at this time (Filene et al., 2013; Goyal et al., 2013; McFarlane et al., 2010; Olds et al., 1994; Sweet & Appelbaum, 2004). Most home visiting programs are evidence-*informed* (Lutzker & Edwards, 2009), but they lack consistent and rigorous outcome data to document their true effectiveness. This is especially concerning given that most maltreatment victims are suffering from neglect at the time of their death. It speaks to the importance of being able to design and implement effective programs that focus on caregivers' ability to supervise and to keep children safe in their homes.

References

Agran, P. D. D. (1991). Unsupervised children in vehicles: A risk for pediatric trauma. *Pediatrics, 87*(1), 70.

Altman, R. L., Canter, J., Patrick, P. A., Daley, N., Butt, N. K., & Brand, D. A. (2011). Parent education by maternity nurses and prevention of abusive head trauma. *Pediatrics, 128*(5), e1164–e1172. doi:10.1542/peds.2010-3260.

American Academy of Pediatrics. (2009). *Abusive head trauma: A new name for shaken baby syndrome*. Retrieved November 16, 2014, from http://www.aap.org/en-us/about-the-aap/aap-press-room/Pages/Abusive-Head-Trauma-A-New-Name-for-Shaken-Baby-Syndrome.aspx

American Academy of Pediatrics. (2011). *Policy statement – SIDS and other sleep-related infant deaths: Expansion of recommendations for a safe infant sleeping environment*. Retrieved January 24, 2015, from http://pediatrics.aappublications.org/content/early/2011/10/12/peds.2011-2284.full.pdf

Armagost, S. (2001). An innocent mistake or criminal conduct: Children dying of hyperthermia in hot vehicles. *Hamline Journal of Public Law & Policy, 23*(1), 109–144.

Barkin, S., & Gelberg, L. (1999). Sink or swim—Clinicians don't often counsel on drowning prevention. *Pediatrics, 104*(Supplement 6), 1217–1219.

Barnett, E. R., Rosenberg, H. J., Rosenberg, S. D., Osofsky, J. D., & Wolford, G. L. (2014). Innovations in practice: Dissemination and implementation of child–parent psychotherapy in rural public health agencies. *Child and Adolescent Mental Health, 19*(3), 215–218.

Barr, R. G. (2012). Preventing abusive head trauma resulting from a failure of normal interaction between infants and their caregivers. *Proceedings of the National Academy of Sciences of the United States of America, 109*(Suppl 2), 17294–17301. doi:10.1073/pnas.1121267109.

Barr, R. G., Barr, M., Fujiwara, T., Conway, J., Catherine, N., & Brant, R. (2009). Do educational materials change knowledge and behaviour about crying and shaken baby syndrome? A randomized controlled trial. *Canadian Medical Association Journal, 180*(7), 727–733.

References

Barr, R. G., Rivara, F. P., Barr, M., Cummings, P., Taylor, J., Lengua, L. J., et al. (2009). Effectiveness of educational materials designed to change knowledge and behaviors regarding crying and Shaken-Baby Syndrome in mothers of newborns: A randomized, controlled trial. *Pediatrics, 123*(3), 972–980.

Barth, R. P. (2009). Preventing child abuse and neglect with parent training: Evidence and opportunities. *The Future of Children, 19*(2), 95–118.

Bidgood, B. A., & van de Sande, A. (1990). Home-based programming for a child welfare clientele. In M. Rothery & G. Cameron (Eds.), *Child maltreatment: Expanding our concept of helping* (pp. 107–125). Hillsdale, NJ: Lawrence Erlbaum Associates, Inc.

Bodenmann, G., Cina, A., Ledermann, T., & Sanders, M. R. (2008). The efficacy of the Triple P-Positive Parenting Program in improving parenting and child behavior: A comparison with two other treatment conditions. *Behaviour Research and Therapy, 46*(4), 411–427.

Canellos, P. S. (2003, August 28). Vt. program delivers dose of Dr. Dean. *Boston Globe*. Retrieved from http://www.boston.com/news/nation/articles/2003/08/28/vt_program_delivers_dose_of_dr_dean/

Carbaugh, S. F. (2004). Understanding shaken baby syndrome. *Advances in Neonatal Care, 4*(2), 105–117. doi:10.1016/j.adnc.2004.1001.1004.

Centers for Disease Control & Prevention. (2012). *Heads up: Prevent shaken baby syndrome. Injury prevention & control: Traumatic brain injury*. Retrieved November 16, 2014, from http://www.cdc.gov/concussion/HeadsUp/sbs.html

Centers for Disease Control & Prevention. (2014a). *Essentials for childhood: Steps to create safe, stable, nurturing relationships and environments*. Retrieved December 16, 2014, from http://www.cdc.gov/violenceprevention/pdf/essentials_for_childhood_framework.pdf

Centers for Disease Control & Prevention. (2014b). *Preventing child maltreatment: Program activities guide*. Retrieved January 3, 2015, from http://www.cdc.gov/violenceprevention/pdf/cm_prog_activities_guide-a.pdf

Centers for Disease Control & Prevention. (2014c). *Unintentional drowning: Get the facts*. Retrieved December 15, 2014, from http://www.cdc.gov/homeandrecreationalsafety/watersafety/waterinjuries-factsheet.html

Centers for Disease Control & Prevention. (n.d.). *Preventing shaken baby syndrome: A guide for health departments and community-based organizations Heads Up*. Atlanta, GA: Centers for Disease Control & Prevention.

Chaffin, M. (2004). Is it time to rethink healthy start/healthy families? *Child Abuse & Neglect, 28*(6), 589–595. doi: http://dx.doi.org/10.1016/j.chiabu.2004.04.004.

Chaffin, M., Funderburk, B., Bard, D., Valle, L. A., & Gurwitch, R. (2011). A combined motivation and parent-child interaction therapy package reduces child welfare recidivism in a randomized dismantling field trial. *Journal of Consulting and Clinical Psychology, 79*(1), 84–95. doi:10.1037/a0021227.

Chaffin, M., Silovsky, J. F., Funderburk, B., Valle, L. A., Brestan, E. V., Balachova, T., … Bonner, B. L. (2004). Parent-child interaction therapy with physically abusive parents: Efficacy for reducing future abuse reports. *Journal of Consulting and Clinical Psychology, 72*(3), 500–510. doi:10.1037/0022-006x.72.3.500.

Collins, J. M. (2006). Crime and parenthood: The uneasy case for prosecuting negligent parents. *Northwestern University Law Review, 100*(2), 807–856.

Covington, T. (2013). The public health approach for understanding and preventing child maltreatment: A brief review of the literature and a call to action. *Child Welfare, 92*(2), 21–39.

Damashek, A., Drass, S., & Bonner, B. L. (2014). Child maltreatment fatalities related to inadequate caregiver supervision. *Journal of Interpersonal Violence, 29*(11), 1987–2001.

de Graaf, I., Speetjens, P., Smit, F., de Wolff, M., & Tavecchio, L. (2008). Effectiveness of the Triple P Positive Parenting Program on parenting: A meta-analysis. *Family Relations: An Interdisciplinary Journal of Applied Family Studies, 57*(5), 553–566.

Dell'Antonia, K. (2011, December 6). A campaign against bed sharing. *The New York Times*. Retrievedfromhttp://parenting.blogs.nytimes.com/2011/12/06/a-controversial-campaign-against-co-sleeping/?_r=0

Dias, M. S., Smith, K., DeGuehery, K., Mazur, P., Li, V., & Shaffer, M. L. (2005). Preventing abusive head trauma among infants and young children: A Hospital-Based, Parent Education Program. *Pediatrics, 115*(4), e470–e477.

Douglas, E. M. (2005). Child maltreatment fatalities: What do we know, what have we done and where do we go from here? In K. Kendall-Tackett & S. Gaicomoni (Eds.), *Child victimization* (pp. 4.1–4.18). Kingston, NJ: Civic Research Institute.

Douglas, E. M. (2015). Using theory to examine fatal child maltreatment among a sample of children known to child protective services. *Journal of Public Child Welfare, 9*(3), 217–235.

Douglas, E. M., & Cunningham, J. M. (2008). Recommendations from child fatality review teams: Results of a US nationwide exploratory study concerning maltreatment fatalities and social service delivery. *Child Abuse Review, 17*(5), 331–351. doi:10.1002/car.1044.

Drazen, S. M., & Haust, M. (1993). Raising reading readiness in low-income children by Parent Education. Draft.

Duggan, A., Caldera, D., Rodriguez, K., Burrell, L., Rohde, C., & Crowne, S. S. (2007). Impact of a statewide home visiting program to prevent child abuse. *Child Abuse & Neglect, 31*(8), 801–827.

Duggan, A., McFarlane, E., Fuddy, L., Burrell, L., Higman, S. M., Windham, A., et al. (2004). Randomized trial of a statewide home visiting program: impact in preventing child abuse and neglect. *Child Abuse & Neglect, 28*(6), 597–622. doi: http://dx.doi.org/10.1016/j.chiabu.2003.08.007.

Dumont, K., Kirkland, K., Mitchell-Herzfeld, S., Ehrhard-Dietzel, S., Lee, E., Layne, C., et al. (2010). *A randomized trial of Healthy Families New York (HFNY): Does home visiting prevent child maltreatment?* Rensselaer, NY: New York State Office of Children & Family Services and Albany.

Durfee, M., Durfee, D. T., & West, M. P. (2002). Child fatality review: An international movement. *Child Abuse & Neglect, 26*, 619–636.

Eckenrode, J. (2000). What works in nurse home visiting programs. In M. P. Kluger, G. Alexander, & P. A. Curtis (Eds.), *What works in child welfare* (pp. 35–43). Washington, DC: Child Welfare League of America.

Edwards, A., Lutzker, J. R., Self-Brown, S., & Whitaker, D. (2012). SafeCare: Addressing child maltreatment from a public health perspective. In J. R. Lutzker & J. Merrick (Eds.), *Applied public health: Examining multifaceted social or ecological problems and child maltreatment* (pp. 119–132). Hauppauge, NY: Nova Biomedical Books.

Edwards-Gaura, A., Whitaker, D. J., Lutzker, J. R., Self-Brown, S., & Lewis, E. (2012). SafeCare: Application of an evidence-based program to prevent child maltreatment. In A. Rubin (Ed.), *Programs and interventions for maltreated children and families at risk* (pp. 259–272). Hoboken, NJ: Wiley.

Fein, L. G. (1979). Can child fatalities, end product child abuse, be prevented? *Children and Youth Services Review, 1*, 31–53.

Fergusson, D. M., Horwood, J., & Ridder, E. M. (2005). *Early Start evaluation report*. Retrieved January 24, 2015, from http://www.otago.ac.nz/christchurch/otago014859.pdf

Filene, J. H., Kaminski, J. W., Valle, L. A., & Cachat, P. (2013). Components associated with home visiting program outcomes: A meta-analysis. *Pediatrics, 132*(Supplement 2), S100–S109. doi:10.1542/peds.2013-1021H.

Fletcher, R., Freeman, E., & Matthey, S. (2011). The impact of behavioural parent training on fathers' parenting: A meta-analysis of the Triple P-Positive Parenting Program. *Fathering: A Journal of Theory, Research, and Practice about Men as Fathers, 9*(3), 291–312.

Funderburk, B. W., & Elherg, S. (2011). Parent-child interaction therapy. In J. C. Norcross, G. R. VandenBos, & D. K. Freedheim (Eds.), *History of psychotherapy: Continuity and change* (2nd ed.). Washington, DC: American Psychological Association.

Gardner, R., Hodson, D., Churchill, G., & Cotmore, R. (2014). Transporting and implementing the SafeCare® home-based programme for parents, designed to reduce and mitigate the effects of child neglect: An initial progress report. *Child Abuse Review, 23*(4), 297–303.

Gelles, R. J. (1996). *The book of David: How preserving families can cost children's lives*. New York, NY: Basic Books.

References

Gershater-Molko, R. M., Lutzker, J. R., & Wesch, D. (2002). Using recidivism to evaluate project safecare: Teaching bonding, safety, and health care skills to parents. *Child Maltreatment, 7*(3), 277.

Goyal, N. K., Teeters, A., & Ammerman, R. T. (2013). Home visiting and outcomes of preterm infants: A systematic review. *Pediatrics, 132*(3), 502–516. doi:10.1542/peds.2013-0077.

Green, A. H., Power, E., Steinbook, B., & Gaines, R. (1981). Factors associated with successful and unsuccessful intervention with child abusive families. *Child Abuse & Neglect, 5*(1), 45–52.

Greenland, C. (1989). *Preventing CAN deaths: An international study of deaths due to child abuse and neglect.* London, UK: Routledge & Kegan Paul.

Guard, A., & Gallagher, S. S. (2005). Heat related deaths to young children in parked cars: An analysis of 171 fatalities in the United States, 1995–2002. *Injury Prevention, 11*(1), 33–37. doi:10.1136/ip.2003.004044.

Guterman, N. B. (1999). Enrollment strategies in early home visitation to prevent physical child abuse and neglect and the 'Universal versus targeted' debate: A meta-analysis of population-based and screening-based programs. *Child Abuse & Neglect, 23*(9), 863–890.

Guterman, N. B. (2001). *Stopping child maltreatment before it starts: Emerging horizons in early home visitation services.* Thousand Oaks, CA: Sage.

Halpern, R. (1986). Home-based early intervention: Dimensions of current practice. *Child Welfare: Journal of Policy, Practice, and Program, 65*(4), 387–398.

Heinrichs, N., Kliem, S., & Hahlweg, K. (2014). Four-year follow-up of a randomized controlled trial of Triple P group for parent and child outcomes. *Prevention Science, 15*(2), 233–245.

Kitzman, H., Olds, D. L., Henderson, C. R., Jr., Cole, R., Tatelbaum, R., McConnochie, K. M., … Hanks, C. (1997). Effect of prenatal and infancy home visitation by nurses on pregnancy outcomes, childhood injuries, and repeated childbearing. A randomized controlled trial. *JAMA, 278*(8), 644–652.

Lee, L. K., & Thompson, K. M. (2007). Parental survey of beliefs and practices about bathing and water safety and their children: Guidance for drowning prevention. *Accident Analysis and Prevention, 39*(1), 58–62.

Lowell, D. I., Carter, A. S., Godoy, L., Paulicin, B., & Briggs-Gowan, M. J. (2011). A randomized controlled trial of child FIRST: A comprehensive home-based intervention translating research into early childhood practice. *Child Development, 82*(1), 193–208. doi:10.1111/j.1467-8624.2010.01550.x.

Lutzker, J. R., & Edwards, A. (2009). SafeCare®: Towards wide-scale implementation of a child maltreatment prevention program. *International Journal of Child Health and Human Development, 2*(1), 7–15.

MacLeod, J., & Nelson, G. (2000). Programs for the promotion of family wellness and the prevention of child maltreatment: A meta-analytic review. *Child Abuse & Neglect, 24*(9), 1127–1149.

Marcenko, M. O., & Spence, M. (1994). Home visitation services for at-risk pregnant and postpartum women: A randomized trial. *American Journal of Orthopsychiatry, 64*(3), 468–478.

Mazzucchelli, T. G., & Sanders, M. R. (2011). Preventing behavioural and emotional problems in children who have a developmental disability: A public health approach. *Research in Developmental Disabilities, 32*(6), 2148–2156.

McFarlane, E., Burrell, L., Fuddy, L., Tandon, D., Derauf, D. C., Leaf, P., et al. (2010). Association of home visitors' and mothers' attachment style with family engagement. *Journal of Community Psychology, 38*(5), 541–556. doi:10.1002/jcop.20380.

McLaren, C., Null, J., & Quinn, J. (2005). Heat stress from enclosed vehicles: Moderate ambient temperatures cause significant temperature rise in enclosed vehicles. *Pediatrics, 116*(1), e109–e112. doi:10.1542/peds.2004-2368.

Morawska, A., Sanders, M., Goadby, E., Headley, C., Hodge, L., McAuliffe, C., … Anderson, E. (2011). Is the Triple P-Positive Parenting Program acceptable to parents from culturally diverse backgrounds? *Journal of Child and Family Studies, 20*(5), 614–622.

Morawska, A., Tometzki, H., & Sanders, M. R. (2014). An evaluation of the efficacy of a Triple P-Positive Parenting Program podcast series. *Journal of Developmental and Behavioral Pediatrics, 35*(2), 128–137.

Morrongiello, B. A., Corbett, M., McCourt, M., & Johnston, N. (2006). Understanding unintentional injury risk in young children II. The contribution of caregiver supervision, child attributes, and parent attributes. *Journal of Pediatric Psychology, 31*(6), 540–551.

Morrongiello, B. A., Sandomierski, M., & Spence, J. R. (2014). Changes over swim lessons in parents' perceptions of children's supervision needs in drowning risk situations: "His swimming has improved so now he can keep himself safe". *Health Psychology, 33*(7), 608–615. doi:10.1037/a0033881.

National Conference of State Legislatures. (2014, January). *Shaken baby syndrome prevention legislation.* From http://www.ncsl.org/research/human-services/shaken-baby-syndrome-prevention-legislation.aspx

National Highway Traffic Safety Administration. (n.d.). *Heatstroke: Prevent child heatstroke in cars. Parents central – From car seats to car keys: Keeping kids safe.* Retrieved December 14, 2014, from http://icsw.nhtsa.gov/safercar/parents/heatstroke.htm

New York City Administration for Children's Services. (2002). *Mayor Michael R. Bloomberg marks child abuse awareness month with public education campaign to reduce shaken baby syndrome.* Retrieved December 4, 2014, from http://www.nyc.gov/html/acs/html/pr_archives/pr02_04_23.shtml

New York State Office of Children and Family Services. (2014). *OCFS promotes safe sleep campaign in areas across New York state.* Retrieved December 27, 2014, from http://ocfs.ny.gov/main/view_article.asp?ID=974

North Carolina Child Fatality Task Force. (2014a). *2012 Child deaths in North Carolina: Trend in rate of child deaths 1991–2012, ages birth through 17 years.* Retrieved December 27, 2014, from http://www.ncleg.net/DocumentSites/Committees/NCCFTF/ReportsandData/2012ChildDeathChart.pdf

North Carolina Child Fatality Task Force. (2014b). *Child death rate down 45% since inception of the Child Fatality Task Force.* Retrieved December 27, 2014, from http://www.ncleg.net/DocumentSites/Committees/NCCFTF/Homepage/

Nurse-Family Partnership. (2014). *Nurse-Family Partnership overview.* Retrieved January 3, 2015, from http://www.nursefamilypartnership.org/assets/PDF/Fact-sheets/NFP_Overview.aspx

Ohio Department of Health. (2014a). *Safe sleep facts.* Retrieved January 24, 2015, from http://www.odh.ohio.gov/features/odhfeatures/SafeSleep/SafeSleepFacts.aspx

Ohio Department of Health. (2014b). *Sleep-related infant deaths. Maternal and Child Health: Early Childhood.* Retrieved January 24, 2015, from http://www.odh.ohio.gov/~/media/ODH/ASSETS/Files/datastatistics/maternal and child health/ec_Sleeprelatedinfant.ashx

Olds, D. L. (2006). The nurse–family partnership: An evidence-based preventive intervention. *Infant Mental Health Journal, 27*(1), 5–25. doi:10.1002/imhj.20077.

Olds, D. L., Eckenrode, J., Henderson, C. R., Jr., et al. (1997). Long-term effects of home visitation on maternal life course and child abuse and neglect: Fifteen-year follow-up of a randomized trial. *JAMA, 278*(8), 637–643. doi:10.1001/jama.1997.03550080047038.

Olds, D. L., Henderson, C. R., Chamberlin, R., & Tatelbaum, R. (1986). Preventing child abuse and neglect: A randomized trial of nurse home visitation. *Pediatrics, 78*(1), 65–78.

Olds, D. L., Henderson, C. R., & Kitzman, H. (1994). Does prenatal and infancy nurse home visitation have enduring effects on qualities of parental caregiving and child health at 25 to 50 months of life? *Pediatrics, 93*(1), 89–98.

Olds, D. L., & Kitzman, H. (1993). Review of research on home visiting for pregnant women and parents of young children. *The Future of Children, 3*(3), 53–92.

Olds, D. L., Kitzman, H., Knudtson, M. D., Anson, E., Smith, J. A., & Cole, R. (2014). Effect of home visiting by nurses on maternal and child mortality: Results of a 2-decade follow-up of a randomized clinical trial. *JAMA Pediatrics, 168*(9), 800–806. doi:10.1001/jamapediatrics.2014.472.

Oliver, M. (2014, September 3). Scrutinizing child deaths in Alabama is paying off, state says. *AL.com.* Retrieved from http://www.al.com/news/index.ssf/2014/09/scrutinizing_child_deaths_in_a.html

Peterson, L. (1994). Child injury and abuse-neglect: Common etiologies, challenges, and courses toward prevention. *Current Directions in Psychological Science, 3*(4), 116–120.

Poole, M. K., Seal, D. W., & Taylor, C. A. (2014). A systematic review of universal campaigns targeting child physical abuse prevention. *Health Education Research, 29*(3), 388–432. doi:10.1093/her/cyu012.

Prinz, R. J., Sanders, M. R., Shapiro, C. J., Whitaker, D. J., & Lutzker, J. R. (2009). Population-based prevention of child maltreatment: The U.S. triple P system population trial. *Prevention Science, 10*(1), 1–12.

Reese, L. S., Heiden, E. O., Kim, K. Q., & Yang, J. (2014). Evaluation of period of PURPLE crying, an abusive head trauma prevention program. *Journal of Obstetric, Gynecologic, and Neonatal Nursing: JOGNN/NAACOG, 43*(6), 752–761.

Runyan, D. K., Hennink-Kaminski, H. J., Zolotor, A. J., Barr, R. G., Murphy, R. A., Barr, M., … Nocera, M. (2009). Designing and testing a shaken baby syndrome prevention program—The Period of PURPLE Crying: Keeping babies safe in North Carolina. *Social Marketing Quarterly, 15*(4), 2–24.

Russell, B. S., Trudeau, J., & Britner, P. A. (2008). Intervention type matters in primary prevention of abusive head injury: Event history analysis results. *Child Abuse & Neglect, 32*(10), 949–957.

Sacramento County Child Death Review Team. (2012). *A twenty year analysis of child death data, 1990–2009*. Sacramento County, CA: Sacramento County Child Death Review Team.

Safe Kids Worldwide. (2014). *New study: 14% of parents say they have left a child alone inside parked vehicle despite the risks of heatstroke*. Retrieved December 14, 2014, from http://www.safekids.org/press-release/new-study-14-parents-say-they-have-left-child-alone-inside-parked-vehicle-despite

Sanders, M. (1999). Triple P-Positive Parenting Program: Towards an empirically validated multi-level parenting and family support strategy for the prevention of behavior and emotional problems in children. *Clinical Child and Family Psychology Review, 2*(2), 71–90. doi:10.1023/A:1021843613840.

Sanders, M., & Pidgeon, A. (2011). The role of parenting programmes in the prevention of child maltreatment. *Australian Psychologist, 46*(4), 199–209.

Sanders, M. R. (2012). Development, evaluation, and multinational dissemination of the Triple P-Positive Parenting Program. *Annual Review of Clinical Psychology, 8*, 345–379.

Sanders, M. R., Dittman, C. K., Farruggia, S. P., & Keown, L. J. (2014). A comparison of online versus workbook delivery of a self-help positive parenting program. *The Journal of Primary Prevention, 35*(3), 125–133.

Sanders, M. R., & Kirby, J. N. (2014). A public-health approach to improving parenting and promoting children's well-being. *Child Development Perspectives, 8*(4), 250–257.

Sanders, M. R., Kirby, J. N., Tellegen, C. L., & Day, J. J. (2014). The Triple P-Positive Parenting Program: A systematic review and meta-analysis of a multi-level system of parenting support. *Clinical Psychology Review, 34*(4), 337–357.

Sanders, M. R., Pidgeon, A. M., Gravestock, F., Connors, M. D., Brown, S., & Young, R. W. (2004). Does parental attributional retraining and anger management enhance the effects of the Triple P-Positive Parenting Program with parents at risk of child maltreatment? *Behavior Therapy, 35*(3), 513–535.

Shanahan, M., Fleming, P., Nocera, M., Sullivan, K., Murphy, R., & Zolotor, A. (2014). Process evaluation of a statewide abusive head trauma prevention program. *Evaluation and Program Planning, 47*, 18–25. doi:10.1016/j.evalprogplan.2014.07.002.

Silovsky, J. F., Bard, D., Chaffin, M., Hecht, D., Burris, L., Owora, A., … Lutzker, J. (2011). Prevention of child maltreatment in high-risk rural families: A randomized clinical trial with child welfare outcomes. *Children and Youth Services Review, 33*(8), 1435–1444. doi:10.1016/j.childyouth.2011.04.023.

Simon, H. K., Tamura, T., & Colton, K. (2003). Reported level of supervision of young children while in the bathtub. *Ambulatory Pediatrics: The Official Journal of the Ambulatory Pediatric Association, 3*(2), 106–108.

Smith, K. M., & deGuehery, K. A. (2008). Shaken baby syndrome education program: Nurses making a difference. *MCN. The American Journal of Maternal Child Nursing, 33*(6), 371–375. doi:10.1097/01.NMC.0000341258.26169.d4.

Starfield, B., Hyde, J., Gérvas, J., & Heath, I. (2008). The concept of prevention: A good idea gone astray? *Journal of Epidemiology and Community Health, 62*(7), 580–583. doi:10.1136/jech.2007.071027.

Starling, S. P., & Holden, J. R. (1995). Abusive head trauma: The relationship of perpetrators to their victims. *Pediatrics, 95*, 260–262.

Stephenson, C. (2011, November 16). Milwaukee co-sleeping ad stirs nationwide debate. *Journal Sentinel*. Retrieved from http://www.jsonline.com/news/milwaukee/milwaukee-cosleeping-ad-stirs-nationwide-debate-4m33572-133987863.html

Stewart, T. C., Polgar, D., Gilliland, J., Tanner, D. A., Girotti, M. J., Parry, N., et al. (2011). Shaken baby syndrome and a triple-dose strategy for its prevention. *Journal of Trauma and Acute Care Surgery, 71*(6), 1801–1807, 1810.1097/TA.1800b1013e31823c31484a.

Stoll, B., & Anderson, J. K. (2013). Prevention of abusive head trauma: A literature review. *Pediatric Nursing, 39*(6), 300–308.

Sweet, M. A., & Appelbaum, M. I. (2004). Is home visiting an effective strategy? A meta-analytic review of home visiting programs for families with young children. *Child Development, 75*(5), 1435–1456. doi:10.1111/j.1467-8624.2004.00750.x.

This PSA shows why it's best for babies to sleep alone. (2014, December 6). *The San Francisco Globe*. Retrieved from http://sfglobe.com/2014/12/03/this-psa-shows-why-its-best-for-babies-to-sleep-alone/

Thomas, R., & Zimmer-Gembeck, M. J. (2012). Parent–child interaction therapy: An evidence-based treatment for child maltreatment. *Child Maltreatment, 17*(3), 253–266. doi:10.1177/1077559512459555.

Thomas, R.-G. M. J. (2011). Accumulating evidence for parent-child interaction therapy in the prevention of child maltreatment. *Child Development, 82*(1), 177–192. doi:10.1111/j.1467-8624.2010.01548.x.

Timmer, S. G., Urquiza, A. J., Zebell, N. M., & McGrath, J. M. (2005). Parent-child interaction therapy: Application to maltreating parent-child dyads. *Child Abuse & Neglect, 29*(7), 825–842.

Triple P. (n.d.-a). *Five steps to positive parenting*. Retrieved December 24, 2014, from http://www.triplep-parenting.net/glo-en/positive-parenting/five-steps-to-positive-parenting/

Triple P. (n.d.-b). *Positive parenting program*. Retrieved December 23, 2014, from http://www.triplep-parenting.net/glo-en/triple-p/positive-parenting-program/

Triple P. (n.d.-c). *Triple P – The system explained*. Retrieved December 24, 2014, from http://www.triplep.net/glo-en/the-triple-p-system-at-work/the-system-explained/

U.S. Commission to End Child Abuse and Neglect Fatalities. (2016). *Within our reach: A national strategy to eliminate child abuse and neglect fatalities*. Retrieved from http://www.acf.hhs.gov/programs/cb/resource/cecanf-final-report.

U.S. Department of Health & Human Services. (2013). *HHS announces expansion of Maternal, Infant, and Early Childhood Home Visiting* [Press release]. Retrieved from http://www.hhs.gov/news/press/2013pres/09/20130906a.html

Urquiza, A. J., & McNeil, C. B. (1996). Parent-child interaction therapy: An intensive dyadic intervention for physically abusive families. *Child Maltreatment, 1*(2), 134–144.

Vincent, S. (2010a). *Learning from child deaths and serious abuse*. Edinburgh, UK: Dunedin Academic Press Ltd.

Vincent, S. (2010b). *Preventing child deaths: Learning from review*. Edinburgh, UK: Dunedin Academic Press Ltd.

Watts, E. (2013, February 13). PSA warns parents about baby sleeping dangers. *FOX-5-KVVU-TV*. Retrieved from http://www.fox5vegas.com/story/20808759/psa-warns-parents-about-baby-sleeping-dangers

Whitaker, D. J., Ryan, K. A., Wild, R. C., Self-Brown, S., Lutzker, J. R., Shanley, J. R., … Hodges, A. E. (2012). Initial implementation indicators from a statewide rollout of SafeCare within a child welfare system. *Child Maltreatment, 17*(1), 96–101. doi:10.1177/1077559511430722.

Willheim, E. (2013). Dyadic psychotherapy with infants and young children: Child-parent psychotherapy. *Child and Adolescent Psychiatric Clinics of North America, 22*(2), 215–239.

Wright, B. M. (1986). *Infant Mental Health Journal, 7*(4), 247–263.

Chapter 9
Conclusions and Recommendations Moving Forward in the Arena of Fatal Child Maltreatment

The focus of this final chapter is to bring together themes that have emerged throughout the book, summarize important conclusions, and issue recommendations for change. The field of public health has increasingly adopted child maltreatment as an issue that is worthy of being prevented, given the significant individual and societal-level consequences that are associated with it (Chahine, Pecora, & Sanders, 2013; Gibbs et al., 2013; Leeb, Paulozzi, Melanson, Simon, & Arias, 2008). The three levels of public health prevention have been noted at numerous times throughout this book (especially see Chapters 1 and 8). A comprehensive model of prevention includes the following: (1) defining and monitoring the identified problem; (2) identifying risk and protective factors; (3) providing evidence that the identified problem is linked to poor outcomes; (4) using evidence to develop and test prevention approaches; and (5) ensuring widespread adoption (Covington, 2013; Richmond-Crum, Joyner, Fogerty, Ellis, & Saul, 2013). Despite three decades of effort, time, attention, and resources, we are still in the early stages in each of these areas in the prevention of fatal child maltreatment, (noting, of course, that #3 does not apply since the identified problem and "poor outcome" are one in the same).

9.1 The Need for More and Better Research

I have written about social problems and program and policy responses on a variety of topics and have argued before about the need for more and better research to help us address those problems (Douglas, 2006; Douglas & Hines, 2011; Straus, Douglas, & Medeiros, 2014). Never have I seen an area in the social sciences more deserving of additional research and attention, than fatal child maltreatment. Research has consistently shown that children under age 4 are most at risk, that most children die from neglect, that mothers are most often the perpetrators of child maltreatment fatalities (CMFs), African Americans are more likely to be victims, and that boys are slightly more likely to be victims (Bennett et al., 2006; Damashek, Drass, &

Bonner, 2014; Damashek, Nelson, & Bonner, 2013; Palusci & Covington, 2014; U.S. Department of Health & Human Services, 2015). Finally, the parent-child relationship also appears to be key as a risk factor for a CMF (Chance & Scannapieco, 2002; Douglas, 2013; Fein, 1979; Korbin, 1987, 1998). Beyond this, there is little consistent information about children who die from maltreatment, their caregivers, and what the professionals in their lives have done (or not done) to try to prevent their deaths. At a bare minimum, improving the amount and quality of data or research on CMFs requires the following improvements and changes. In fact, this was a key finding of the final report of the U.S. Commission to End Child Abuse and Neglect Fatalities (2016).

9.1.1 Incidence

Public health approaches indicate that in order to tackle a health problem, we need to know how much the problem occurs and to be able to reliably track changes over time (Covington, 2013). This mandates that we have common definitions and ways of counting the problem. We don't have the ability to do this yet with regard to CMFs. Some studies have attempted to estimate the number of children who die from abuse or neglect by reassessing old child death data using current standards or by using "capture-recapture" methods, which statistically estimates the size of a population (Crume, DiGuiseppi, Byers, Sirotnak, & Garrett, 2002; Herman-Giddens et al., 1999; Klevens & Leeb, 2010; Palusci, Wirtz, & Covington, 2010). This has provided us with sufficient information to know that we are missing many, many instances of CMFs. Clearly, we need a consistent method for categorizing and counting how many children die from abuse and neglect. This is a recommendation that has been made repeatedly by child maltreatment scholars (Centers for Disease Control, 1982; Jason, 1984; McClain, Sacks, Froehlke, & Ewigman, 1993; Putnam-Hornstein, Wood, Fluke, Yoshioka-Maxwell, & Berger, 2013; Schnitzer, Gulino, & Ying-Ying, 2013) and now by the U.S. Commission to End Child Abuse and Neglect Fatalities (2016) as well. It is possible that the new federal legislation which mandates that states provide information on the sources of data that states use and do *not use* to count and report cases of fatal child maltreatment will bring more accurate information on the incidence of CMFs in the United States ("Child and Family Services Improvement and Innovation Act," 2011; National Conference of State Legislatures, 2011).

9.1.2 More Complete Data Sources

We need better and more complete data sources. The National Child Abuse and Neglect Data System (NCANDS) is unique because it collects data from all states on the same variables that come from their child welfare information systems. There are limitations, however. Like all datasets that come from applied settings, it has a significant amount of missing data across all variables in the data file. Further, there has never been a year when all states actually submitted their data, so it is an incomplete picture of child welfare-involved families and services received in the U.S. In the area of CMFs, the type of maltreatment is not *necessarily* the cause of death. It is the type of maltreatment for which the caregivers were substantiated. This type of maltreatment could have been recorded before the child's death or after, depending on when the child came to the attention of the agency. For example, if a parent was substantiated for physical abuse and then her child drown while being unsupervised around water, that record of physical abuse is what stands on the record, not neglect. Further, each annual dataset does not contain information about whether a child was known to the agency before or after the child's death. One can restrict the data to only look at cases where the child was a "prior victim"—in other words, a case that would have previously been substantiated to child protective services. But if the child had been the subject of a report it is impossible to know if that was before or after the death, because there is no date of death that is listed. One can place a special request at the National Data Archive on Child Abuse and Neglect at Cornell University to link together separate annual files over time to see if a case that ended in fatality in one year had been the subject of report in previous years. But, looking at the data file year-by-year, one cannot tell if a report was made before the child died, or if the report that exists was to report that incident of the maltreatment fatality. Because of issues of confidentiality, NCANDS masks the state and county of the CMF victim, which makes it impossible to examine how state or county-level factors might be related to a child's death from abuse or neglect. In order to more fully examine CMFs using the NCANDS data, at a minimum, there should be information about the date that the child died, the type of maltreatment that killed the child, and the relationship between the child and the perpetrator of the fatality. Despite confidentiality concerns, knowing the state in which a child died would allow researchers to examine how CMFs might be related to state funding, child welfare workforce issues, and changes in child welfare policy and practice. Finally, national-level data on CMFs should be housed at a national archive, such as the one at Cornell, so that questions can be assessed by researchers far and wide.

9.1.3 Risk Factors

We have limited knowledge about what risk factors distinguish fatal from non-fatal maltreatment. When I talk to knowledgeable audiences about risk factors for fatal child maltreatment, I am inevitably asked, "Those are risk factors for abuse and neglect that does not end in death. What's the difference?" In truth, we don't know. It may not be one single factor, but might be a combination of risk factors—something which has been examined by only a handful of studies (Douglas, 2015; Yampolskaya, Greenbaum, & Berson, 2009). The field does not yet know what is the tipping point of when a family, a child, or a case moves from being an example of non-fatal maltreatment into the red zone of being at-risk for fatality. This is obviously crucially important information for the fields of child welfare, health, and social services.

How are children and their families who are known to child protective services before they die distinct from those who are unknown? There has been no research conducted on this topic so far and NCANDS does not allow for this type of examination. Studies on CMF victims do include cases that were both known and unknown to professional helping groups prior to a child's death, but these two groups of children have yet to be compared. This kind of information could help expand outreach to children and families who need support and increase reporting to child protective services for children who are at-risk of death.

There are a host of risk factors for non-fatal child maltreatment that have not been fully investigated with regard to fatal maltreatment, including: family social isolation, physical isolation, parental substance use, children's living arrangement, violence within the family (including partner violence), housing stability, parent socioeconomic level, and the parent-child relationship, although there are likely more. There is some emerging research on the distinguishing risk factors for an abuse death versus a neglect death (Damashek et al., 2013; Douglas, 2014). We need more of this research, because abuse and neglect are distinct forms of maltreatment, even though we often treat them as one (Anderson, Ambrosino, Valentine, & Lauderdale, 1983; Brewster et al., 1998; Crume et al., 2002; Jenny & Isaac, 2006; Johnson, 2000). More accurate information on their distinguishing characteristics could help prevent CMFs.

9.1.4 CMFs and Helping Professions

Did a professional try to intervene before a child died? If so, what was done? What was not done? I have done a small bit of work on the services that families received prior to a child's death (Douglas, 2013, 2016; Douglas & Mohn, 2014), but it is only the beginning of work that needs to be done in this area. The field needs more of this information so that we can better understand if families where children die are not receiving services at all, are receiving too few services, incorrect services, too few of the right services, or services of poor quality. These are all questions that we need to be able to answer in our attempt to prevent future deaths. Today, however, these remain question marks.

Most of the research concerning fatal child maltreatment and professionals has focused on child welfare professionals, but CMF victims come into contact with many other professionals prior to their death: judges, pediatricians, visiting home nurses, and other family support workers. For example, what if a judge is not convinced of a potential threat to a child and returns the child to his or her parents, despite the concerns of child welfare workers? And, what if that child then dies? That case will likely fall at the feet of the child welfare agency, despite their efforts to protect the child. What if physicians fail to detect symptoms of physical child abuse and a child is sent home from the hospital with parents who perpetrate more violence against a child who eventually dies? I once read a case where a family support worker failed to recognize symptoms of SBS and instead thought that an infant simply had a cold or the flu. We don't how these professionals are trained to recognize risk factors for CMFs, the actions that they take when encountered with such risk factors, and the like. This is an area that is ripe for future research.

9.2 What's Working?

Before I discuss what's working, let's quickly review what I've covered in this book. Multidisciplinary child death review teams (CDRTs) have been implemented across the country to review and identify problems associated with children's deaths in an attempt to prevent more in the future. Every state in the Union has passed a law that allows parents to legally relinquish their (relatively) new infants without fear of criminal consequences. The criminal justice system has passed laws that allow parents who actively or passively kill children to be punished more harshly than under older laws. In the area of prevention, there are a host of approaches, including shaken baby prevention programs, public education campaigns about the dangers of leaving children unsupervised in cars, around water, etc., early home visiting programs to support families with very young children, and general parent education or training programs to prevent maltreatment, but primarily physical abuse. I hope that this book has illuminated the tremendous efforts that many different fields have taken to address CMFs, from many different angles.

What is most troubling about these efforts is that we do not know how well they work. We know that CDRTs have allowed us to bring multiple players to the table to talk about the circumstances under which children die, which causes of deaths should be ruled abuse or neglect, and to collect data on the child, family, and household characteristics of the victims (American Academy of Pediatrics, 2010; Covington, 2011; Durfee, Durfee, & West, 2002; Webster, Schnitzer, Jenny, Ewigman, & Alario, 2003). There is very little documented evidence of the change that results from these discussions (Palusci, Yager, & Covington, 2010). Based on my experience of working for such a team, these multidisciplinary discussions lead to informal changes in practice or operations for professionals working with vulnerable children and their families. Without knowing what are those changes, however, it is difficult to determine the magnitude of their impact. This is important because CDRTs are resource intensive, especially in the form of professionals' time. Do we know more about the risk factors that children face with regard to fatalities because of CDRTs? I would say, yes. Are more children appropriately identified as having died from abuse or neglect than before CDRTs were in existence? I would say, yes. And, do fewer children die because of the activities of CDRTs? As of now, there is no direct evidence that this is the case. It is possible that CDRT activities have led to increased attention to infant deaths, which have prompted many of the initiatives to prevent SBS, some of which have been effective and resulted in fewer cases of

SBS. Without more research, one can only speculate regarding the effectiveness of CDRTs, based on what evidence—both official and anecdotal—is available.

Newspapers across the United States document instances where safe haven laws have permitted parent to legally relinquish live infants into the care and protection of a designated professional (Domash, Gallucci, & Twarowski, 2010; Ontiveros, 2014; Rizzi & Hinko, 2011). Would that child have otherwise been abandoned and died? Possibly so. Without the presence of safe haven laws, would that parent have worked with an adoption agency to arrange for a traditional adoption? Perhaps. Or, without a safe haven option, would that parent have kept the child and s/he would have wound up in the child welfare system? Maybe. It's just not possible to tell. We cannot concretely say that safe haven laws prevent the deaths of infants. We can say that babies are turned over through the safe haven system in every state. We do not know what would have happened to those children otherwise and without a national registry, we don't know how many children are relinquished in this manner (Oberman, 2008). But, comparatively speaking, safe haven laws are relatively inexpensive and we do know that the safe haven approach provides a system for parents to relinquish live infants, free, and safe from harm, for both the infants and relinquishers. At the same time, these laws do not help to prevent unwanted pregnancies, they do not provide a way for infants who are later adopted to have a connection to their families of origin, and we cannot deny that despite the presence of these laws, infants continue to be discarded and to die.

Historically, the perpetrators of fatal child maltreatment spent little-to-no time in jail (Commonwealth of Virginia Department for Children, 1990; United States Advisory Board on Child Abuse and Neglect, 1995). Now, most states in the country have passed laws which allow them to more harshly prosecute perpetrators if the victims are considered to be a minor and suffered maltreatment (National Center for the Prosecution of Child Abuse, 2013; Phipps, 1999). Only a few investigations have been conducted into whether perpetrators of child homicide victims spend more or less time in jail, compared with perpetrators of adult homicide victims (Augé & Mitchell, 2012; Hewes, Keenan, McDonnell, Dudley, & Herman, 2011). Are these laws meant to deter caregivers from killing children or to respond to a call for social justice that demands harsher penalties when children are victims? Probably both. But, at the present time, we have no idea if the laws that are on the books are being implemented in the field or if they act as a deterrent for caregivers. That said, I wouldn't necessarily recommend repeal these laws, because with the exception of costs associated with increased jail time, these laws do not appear to be expensive and at present, there is no evidence that they are harmful.

Finally, we turn to prevention (the topic of the child welfare profession deserves its own separate section). The story here is a little more complex. In short, there are very few educational efforts to explicitly prevent the deaths of children. If this is a goal, then prevention programs addressing shaken baby syndrome (SBS) come the closest to meeting this goal. Further, if the appropriate programs are selected and implemented, there is evidence that fewer children sustain head injuries which often lead to death (Dias et al., 2005). There are public service announcements that focus on supervising children in a variety of settings, but they have not been evaluated and so we do not know whether they are effective. Finally, we come to programs that prevent child maltreatment, in general. The programs showing some effectiveness for preventing or reducing child maltreatment so far are First CHILD, Nurse-Family Partnership, an augmented version of SafeCare, Triple P, and Parent-Child Interaction Therapy. These programs primarily focus on preventing physical abuse and they are widely considered promising programs (Chaffin et al., 2004; Olds, Eckenrode, Henderson et al., 1997; Poole, Seal, & Taylor, 2014; Prinz, Sanders, Shapiro, Whitaker, & Lutzker, 2009). None have not been used to test their ability to prevent fatalities or risk-factors for specifically CMFs, however. As noted in Chapter 8, the U.S. Commission to End Child Abuse and Neglect Fatalities (2016), heralded the Nurse-Family Partnership as being the only home visiting program that prevents fatalities. It is true that families in the treatment group experienced no fatalities over a 21-year period of time, while nine children from the control group did die from preventable causes (Olds et al., 2014). These deaths were not specific to maltreatment and to endorsement the Nurse-Family Partnership as such is, from my perspective, slightly misleading. Finally, it is important to note that child maltreatment prevention programs have been less successful in preventing neglect, which is the form of maltreatment that most often kills children. It is noteworthy, too, that one member of the U.S. Commission to End Child Abuse and Neglect Fatalities failed to sign their 2016 report, stating that the Commission was encouraging the adoption of programs and services that lack evidence in terms of their effectiveness.

9.3 Child Welfare Profession—Crisis or Crossroads?

Take any day, of any week, in any year, and a child welfare agency somewhere in the United States is in crisis over the death of a child, who was known to the agency before that child died. That is the definition of a crisis and it goes without saying, a tragedy. In such instances, there is often tremendous backlash from the community and the state legislature, like the time that a state legislator in Maine suggested that the Department of Human Services should instead be called the Department of Human *Sacrifice* (Meara, 1999). This kind of crisis can lead to opportunity and that's the way most state agencies try to recover from such disasters—by firing seemingly incompetent staff, changing screening procedures for assessing and responding to cases of child abuse or neglect, bringing in trainers, adopting a new model of child welfare practice, and in the most desperate of times, changing the name of the agency (a notion which I mention in modest jest, even though it is true (Otis, 2014; Pitzl, 2014)). There have recently been several states in crisis, namely—Arizona, Connecticut, Massachusetts, and Florida. Perhaps it is time to take a new look at what is going on in the child welfare profession. I provided some of this information in Chapter 4, but I summarize the content here, along with recommendations for change.

The research that I have conducted shows that child welfare workers are very concerned that a child on his or her caseload may die and that most workers actively assess for factors that they think may lead to a child's death. That said, my research also shows that workers have low levels of knowledge about the known risk factors for fatalities (Douglas, 2012). This reality makes it difficult for workers to do their job. This is an area that must be addressed through training. But, it should not stop with training; this knowledge should be incorporated into their daily work, risk assessments conducted on families, interactions with families, and into conversations that they have with their supervisors. This latter part is especially important because research shows that the relationship that workers have with their supervisors determine their engagement and longevity in the field (Mor Barak, Levin, Nissly, & Lane, 2006; Travis & Mor Barak, 2010).

There is potentially a more fundamental area of concern in child welfare practice: the integration of the strengths-based approach within the child welfare and social service professions (Roose, Roets, & Schiettecat, 2014). I openly state that there is no research to back up these concerns, but my years in and around the field, and anecdotal evidence indicate that this is an area that demands attention so that we can learn more about this practice approach. As I explain in Chapter 4, the child welfare profession has embraced the strengths perspective (Kemp, Marcenko, Lyons, & Kruzich, 2014; Lietz, 2011; Lietz & Rounds, 2009; Mapp, 2002), as a practice approach toward working with families, yet there is little evidence to back up this theoretical orientation (Staudt, Howard, & Drake, 2001). There are two areas that are most concerning. First, there is such a focus on finding strengths in families, that it may divert workers' attention from assessing for or fully conceptualizing when risk is present in a child's life. Second, there is no discussion of what constitutes a strength. When consulting on cases or teaching, I hear stories about workers who identify parent or family characteristics as strengths: "the mother said she wants to go to school," "the father just applied for a job," "the parents just got married," "the family just moved to a new apartment" or "the mother wants her child to be happy." In these circumstances, what is really being described is a "positive element" in a person's life, as opposed to parent or family characteristics that have the ability to act in a protective capacity toward a child. The child welfare profession could benefit from more fully conceptualizing how a strengths approach *works* in the child welfare profession, what *constitutes* a strength, and does focusing on strengths mean *turning away* from risk. Some child welfare agencies assess for "protective capacities" as a proxy for strengths (ACTION for Child Protection, 2010). In this approach, workers assess for specific characteristics that would allow a parent or caregiver to protect a child, for example: "What does the person know about child development?" "What does the person know about parenting?" and "How does the person view child rearing in terms of difficulty, complexity, or challenge?" (p. 3). Although also not the result of rigorous evaluation, it provides workers with concrete characteristics and capacities to assess when working with families (American Psychological Association, 2013; Budd, 2005).

9.4 What if We Focused on the *Fatal* Part of a Child Maltreatment Fatality?

Over the past three decades, there has been a tremendous amount of writing that has focused on preventing fatal child maltreatment. This literature has largely come in one of two forms. The first discusses the tremendous opportunity that CDRTs offer to learn about the circumstances under which children die, child, caregiver, and household characteristics, and where the social welfare/health services systems intervened, if at all (Covington, 2011; Hochstadt, 2006; Onwuachi-Saunders, Forjuoh, West, & Brooks, 1999; Palusci, Yager, & Covington, 2010; Vincent, 2010; Webster et al., 2003; Wirtz, Foster, & Lenart, 2011). The other approach has been to discuss preventing CMFs by focusing on the prevention of child abuse and neglect, in general, or changing the capacity of the child welfare system to respond to maltreatment (Brandon, 2009; Chahine et al., 2013; Covington, 2013; Creighton, 1995; Fein, 1979; Richmond-Crum et al., 2013). What if, instead of trying to prevent maltreatment fatalities by only focusing on the prevention of maltreatment, we also started focusing on what puts children at risk for a fatality? It is true that our knowledge in this area is limited, but it is growing.

My colleague, Melinda Gushwa, at Simmons College, started referring to using a "child maltreatment fatality lens" when we were delivering a training about CMFs to child welfare professionals. *What if we viewed all of our cases through the lens of risk factors for fatalities?* It's an interesting notion. I made a quick reference to this term when I testified in October 2014 before the U.S. Commission to Eliminate Child Abuse & Neglect Fatalities and after my testimony, a service provider who had been sitting in the audience rush up to me, pencil positioned against a writing pad and asked, "What is a 'child maltreatment fatality lens'? I've never heard of that before." Good question.

Using a CMF lens is simply the idea of keeping at the forefront of one's mind a list of known risk factors that place a child at-risk for a CMF. So, for every professional who works with a family or a child, she or he would consider, for example, the age of the child, the type of maltreatment that is being experienced, the parent's expectations about the child's behavior, how many times the family has moved recently, who lives in the house, and so forth. The research that I have conducted shows that workers have low knowledge of risk factors for CMFs (Douglas, 2012). Investigations I have done with colleagues show that we are not adequately preparing professionals about risk factors for CMFs—at least in the child welfare profession (Douglas, Mohn, & Gushwa, 2015; Douglas & Serino, 2013). I'm willing to make the leap that if child welfare professionals are not being trained about risk factors for death, neither are physicians, nurses, psychologists, family support workers, parenting educators, and other social service providers. Instead of putting CMFs on the back burner as an event that rarely happens, what if we moved it to the front burner? What if we made it front-and-center for whenever a child was being examined or a family was being investigated?

What if we took such an approach one step further? Instead of professionals conducting such an evaluation on families, what if professionals also provided information about these risk factors to the caregivers themselves? The education programs that are in place to prevent SBS are tremendous because they have been shown to work (Altman et al., 2011; Dias et al., 2005). What if we took this model and educated parents about how children die, the importance of providing supervision to children and discussed the risk factors in their own lives, while also helping them find ways to reduce those risk factors? This kind of model could be implemented with families in healthcare settings, child protection work, family support services, and through parent education programs.

9.5 Is There Any Good News?

The focus of this book is an ugly one. No one wants to think about children dying, especially not from abuse or neglect, and definitely not at the hands of the people who we hope will love and care for them. On top of this, I have painted a bleak picture of states "throwing" resources at this problem with no documented evidence that what is being done is actually working. Is there any bright spot in this story of doom? I think so.

The brightest spot is not well established, but takes us back to Chapter 2, where I defined fatal child maltreatment and provided rates of victimization over the past two decades. If the reader flips back to that chapter, the bright spot is hidden in Figures 2.1 and 2.2. Information from NCANDS shows that the CMF rate has been increasing for close to two decades. But, the FBI data and the vital statistics data shows a decrease during that same period. Which source is more accurate and why the differences? The latter data sources do not likely have much data on neglect, since a neglect death would have to reach a very high bar in order to be classified as a homicide. Meanwhile, the deaths which have increasingly been getting attention are those that are due to neglect—children left in vehicles, unattended during bath time, children co-sleeping with an intoxicated parent who accidentally smothers the child, or unsupervised children who die in a house fire while their parents gambled the night away in a neighboring town. There is sufficient scientific (Kim, Shapiro-Mendoza, Chu, Camperlengo, & Anderson, 2012; Shapiro-Mendoza, Kimball, Tomashek, Anderson, & Blanding, 2009) and anecdotal evidence to show that the thinking about and approach toward handling these deaths has been changing by child welfare professionals and medical examiners.

These tremendous changes have been taking place at the same time as another unprecedented change in the world of child well-being. The rates of physical and child sexual abuse have been declining since the mid-1990s (Finkelhor & Jones, 2012; Jones & Finkelhor, 2003; Jones, Finkelhor, & Halter, 2006; Jones, Finkelhor, & Kopiec, 2001). There is a well-established set of research which has documented a decline in these two forms of abuse, which has been accompanied by other declines in social problems that are related to and that affect youth (Child Trends, 2014; Finkelhor & Jones, 2006; Martin, Hamilton, Osterman, Curtin, & Matthews, 2013). Neglect, on the other hand, has remained relatively constant (Jones et al., 2006). So, what does this all mean for the rate of CMFs?

Here's what we know to be true: (1) child physical abuse has been on the decline; (2) rates of child neglect have remained relatively flat during this time period; (3) child homicide statistics were also on the decline during this same period; (4) the CMF rate increased over this period; and (5) there were changes in how we approach many causes of child deaths and what was once considered to be unknown or accidental causes of death are now sometimes considered a form of neglect. Given this set of information, I cautiously conclude that there may be good news. The rate of deaths by abuse likely declined and the rate of deaths by neglect likely remained steady, but were more accurately identified, thus making it look like an increase in both the raw numbers and the rate of deaths.

The efficacy of prevention and parenting education programs has been questioned by child welfare professionals for years (Chaffin, 2004; Gelles, 1996). So, the fact that there are programs that are changing parents' behaviors and decreasing the rate of reports to child welfare agencies is a significant achievement. These promising programs, such as First CHILD, Nurse-Family Partnership, SafeCare, Triple P, and Parent-Child Interaction Therapy have specific curricula and should not be generalized to all prevention and parenting education programs. I believe that CDRTs have made a tremendous difference in so many ways, even if they are not well documented. They bring together professionals on a regular basis to discuss common and different approaches to the same cases and over time, the field has gathered more and better data about the cases that are reviewed; further, that data is increasingly comparable between states. This is no small act and has the potential to teach current and future professionals about children who die from maltreatment and their families.

To this list of good news, I will add three additional comments. One, the Baby Safe Haven Alliance helps desperate parents—mostly mothers—find safe solutions for the infants that they cannot or do not want to raise. Two, parents who do not provide medical treatment for their children because of their religious beliefs want what is best for their children, as do most parents. But, the guidance that they have received and their beliefs are out-of-step with our common standards for how to protect and care for children today. Children's Healthcare Is a Legal Duty has made tremendous strides to change religious shield laws and we are seeing some progress in states such as Oregon. There are serious discussions about making similar inroads in Idaho as well (Tilkin, 2013). The final piece of good news is that there is enough concern and activity about CMFs that someone could write an entire book about the various steps that we have taken as a nation—individually and together—to try to prevent future cases of fatal child maltreatment. The recent national legislation to establish the U.S. Commission to Eliminate Child Abuse and Neglect Fatalities is just another example of these efforts, but at a much higher level.

9.6 What Are the Final Recommendations?

Before wrapping up, let's return to the public health model of prevention that started this chapter (Covington, 2013; Richmond-Crum et al., 2013). (1) Defining and monitoring the identified problem—we have made significant progress in this area, but lack common definitions and ways to count CMFs. (2) Identifying risk and protective factors—this is another area where we have made significant gains, but we need better information, especially concerning the distinction between risk factors for fatal and non-fatal child maltreatment. (3) Providing evidence that the identified problem is linked to poor outcomes—this is not applicable since the outcome is the same as the identified problem—fatality. (4) Using evidence to develop and test prevention approaches—we have a long way to go, but the most successful example is SBS prevention programs. (5) Ensure widespread adoption—at this point, we do not have widespread adoption of any program to prevent fatal child maltreatment. We have made significant progress in all of these areas, but we have a long way to go before we turn the tide in the prevention of fatal child maltreatment. The purpose of this book was to evaluate the "state of the field," to determine what is working, what could be changed, and to issue recommendations. This final chapter provides those recommendations, but I close with a bulleted list concerning next steps that I hope will help us to better prevent fatal child maltreatment in the United States.

1. **We need better and more complete data.** This data should provide information about when children entered the child welfare system, definitively indicate whether the child was known to the child welfare system before a death, and the **type of maltreatment that caused the death**. It should provide reliable information about case records and services received. We need detailed information about CMF victims, even if they were unknown prior to the death. National-level data should be housed at a data archive, accessible to qualified researchers in order to advance the state of our knowledge.
2. **We need new research on the intersection of CMFs and many different helping professions**: judges, pediatricians, visiting home nurses, family support workers, and the like. Many helping professionals work with children and families who are at risk for or experiencing abuse or neglect, and we have no understanding of their preparation, knowledge, attitudes, and professional decisions, as it pertains to CMFs.
3. **Child welfare professionals want more training on risk factors** for CMFs and they need it, so let's give it to them. The child welfare system should also define for its workers what constitutes a parent, child or family strength and its ability to serve as a protective factor for a child. Finally, the child welfare system should examine **whether focusing on the strengths** of a family **limits** the profession's ability to simultaneously **assess for risk** and safety.
4. **The outcomes of CDRTs**, the changes that are made as a result of reviews, and the activities that are performed outside of reviews **should be documented** and be made available to members of the teams, state legislatures, and the general

public. There should be some effort to establish if and how CDRT activities result in fewer maltreatment deaths.
5. **There should be a national database which tracks children who are abandoned or safely relinquished through a safe haven program.** This information would be collected at the state level and reported to the federal government on an annual basis. It should provide a clear picture regarding the use of safe haven laws and provide information about the marketing of safe haven laws to specific populations.
6. **All children deserve access to healthcare, regardless of their parents' religious beliefs** and denying children healthcare, for any reason, is a form of neglect. Religious shield laws that allow parents to deny modern medical treatments to their children should be overturned.
7. **The evidence that parenting education and home visiting programs can prevent child abuse and neglect is limited,** especially in the area of neglect, which is the leading cause of both fatal and non-fatal child maltreatment. This is an area that deserves more attention, both in terms of establishing effective programs and then supporting and disseminating programs that effectively reduce child maltreatment.
8. **We should adopt a "child maltreatment fatality lens,"** in which professionals who work with children, especially very young children, assess for known risk factors for fatality and in which we educate parents about the ways that children die and the risk factors for this tragic outcome.

References

ACTION for Child Protection. (2010). *Assessing caregiver protective capacities related to parenting*. Retrieved January 3, 2015, from http://action4cp.org/documents/2010/pdf/June_2010_ Assessing_Caregiver_Protective_Capacities.pdf

Altman, R. L., Canter, J., Patrick, P. A., Daley, N., Butt, N. K., & Brand, D. A. (2011). Parent education by maternity nurses and prevention of abusive head trauma. *Pediatrics, 128*(5), e1164–e1172. doi:10.1542/peds.2010-3260.

American Academy of Pediatrics. (2010). Policy statement—Child fatality review. *Pediatrics, 126*(3), 592–596. doi:10.1542/peds.2010-2006.

American Psychological Association. (2013). Guidelines for psychological evaluation in child protection matters. *American Psychologist, 68*(1), 20–31.

Anderson, R., Ambrosino, R., Valentine, D., & Lauderdale, M. (1983). Child deaths attributed to abuse and neglect: An empirical study. *Children and Youth Services Review, 5*(1), 75–89.

Augé, K., & Mitchell, K. (2012, November 16). Short on justice: Penalties for child deaths less severe than for adults in Colorado. *The Denver Post*. Retrieved from http://www.denverpost.com/failedtodeath/ci_21996958/inequity-exists-length-sentences-deaths-kids-and-adults

Bennett, M. D., Jr., Hall, J., Frazier, L., Jr., Patel, N., Barker, L., & Shaw, K. (2006). Homicide of children aged 0–4 years, 2003–04: Results from the National Violent Death Reporting System. *Injury Prevention: Journal of the International Society for Child and Adolescent Injury Prevention, 12*(Suppl 2), ii39–ii43.

Brandon, M. (2009). Child fatality or serious injury through maltreatment: Making sense of outcomes. *Children and Youth Services Review, 31*(10), 1107–1112.

Brewster, A. L., Nelson, J. P., Hymel, K. P., Colby, D. R., Lucas, D. R., McCanne, T. R., & Milner, J. S. (1998). Victim, perpetrator, family, and incident characteristics of 32 infant maltreatment deaths in the United States Air Force. *Child Abuse & Neglect, 22*(2), 91–101. doi:http://dx.doi.org/10.1016/S0145-2134(97)00132-4.

Budd, K. S. (2005). Assessing parenting capacity in a child welfare context. *Children and Youth Services Review, 27*(4), 429–444. doi: http://dx.doi.org/10.1016/j.childyouth.2004.11.008.

Centers for Disease Control. (1982). Perspectives in disease prevention and health promotion child homicide – United States. *Morbidity and Mortality Weekly Review, 31*, 292–294.

Chaffin, M. (2004). Is it time to rethink Healthy Start/Healthy Families? *Child Abuse & Neglect, 28*(6), 589–595. doi: http://dx.doi.org/10.1016/j.chiabu.2004.04.004.

Chaffin, M., Silovsky, J. F., Funderburk, B., Valle, L. A., Brestan, E. V., Balachova, T., … Bonner, B. L. (2004). Parent-child interaction therapy with physically abusive parents: Efficacy for reducing future abuse reports. *Journal of Consulting and Clinical Psychology, 72*(3): 500–510. doi:10.1037/0022-006x.72.3.500.

Chahine, Z., Pecora, P., & Sanders, D. (2013). Special foreword: Preventing severe maltreatment-related injuries and fatalities: Applying a public health framework and innovative approaches to child protection. *Child Welfare, 92*(2), 13–18.

Chance, T. C., & Scannapieco, M. (2002). Ecological correlates of child maltreatment: Similarities and differences between child fatality and nonfatality cases. *Child and Adolescent Social Work Journal, 19*(2), 139–161.

Child Trends. (2014). *Teen homicide, suicide, and firearm deaths: Indicators on children and youth.* Retrieved January 1, 2015, from http://www.childtrends.org/wp-content/uploads/2014/07/70_Homicide_Suicide_Firearms.pdf

Child and Family Services Improvement and Innovation Act, Pub. L. No. 112–34, H.R. 2883 Stat. (2011).

Commonwealth of Virginia Department for Children. (1990). *Criminal sanctions for child abuse fatalities.* Richmond, VA. Retrieved from http://search.ebscohost.com/login.aspx?direct=true&db=sih&AN=SM126802&site=ehost-live

Covington, T. (2013). The public health approach for understanding and preventing child maltreatment: A brief review of the literature and a call to action. *Child Welfare, 92*(2), 21–39.

Covington, T. M. (2011). The US National Child Death review case reporting system. *Injury Prevention: Journal of the International Society for Child and Adolescent Injury Prevention, 17*(Suppl 1), i34–i37. doi:10.1136/ip.2010.031203.

Creighton, S. J. (1995). Fatal child abuse- How preventable is it? *Child Abuse Review, 4*, 318–328.

Crume, T. L., DiGuiseppi, C., Byers, T., Sirotnak, A. P., & Garrett, C. J. (2002). Underascertainment of child maltreatment fatalities by death certificates, 1990–1998. *Pediatrics, 110*(2), e18.

Damashek, A., Drass, S., & Bonner, B. L. (2014). Child maltreatment fatalities related to inadequate caregiver supervision. *Journal of Interpersonal Violence, 29*(11), 1987–2001.

Damashek, A., Nelson, M. M., & Bonner, B. L. (2013). Fatal child maltreatment: Characteristics of deaths from physical abuse versus neglect. *Child Abuse & Neglect, 37*(10), 735–744. doi: http://dx.doi.org/10.1016/j.chiabu.2013.04.014.

Dias, M. S., Smith, K., DeGuehery, K., Mazur, P., Li, V., & Shaffer, M. L. (2005). Preventing abusive head trauma among infants and young children: A hospital-based, parent education program. *Pediatrics, 115*(4), e470–e477.

Domash, S. F., Gallucci, J., & Twarowski, C. (2010, October 14). *Inside Tim Jaccard's Children of Hope and baby safe haven crusade.* Long Island Press. Retrieved from http://archive.longislandpress.com/2010/10/14/inside-tim-jaccards-children-of-hope-and-baby-safe-haven-crusade/

Douglas, E. M. (2006). *Mending broken families: Social policies for families of divorce–Are they working?* Lanham, MD: Rowman & Littlefield.

Douglas, E. M. (2012). Child welfare workers' training, knowledge, and practice concerns regarding child maltreatment fatalities: An exploratory, multi-state analysis. *Journal of Public Child Welfare, 6*(5), 659–677. doi:10.1080/15548732.2012.723975.

Douglas, E. M. (2013). Case, service and family characteristics of households that experience a child maltreatment fatality in the United States. *Child Abuse Review, 22*(5), 311–326. doi:10.1002/car.2236.

Douglas, E. M. (2014). A comparison of child fatalities by physical abuse versus neglect: Child, family, service, and worker characteristics. *Journal of Social Service Research, 40*(3), 259–273. doi:10.1080/01488376.2014.893948.

Douglas, E. M. (2015). Using theory to examine fatal child maltreatment among a sample of children known to child protective services. *Journal of Public Child Welfare, 9*(3), 217–235. doi:10.1080/15548732.2015.1041668.

Douglas, E. M. (2016). Testing if social services prevent fatal child maltreatment among a sample of children previously known to child protective services. *Child Maltreatment*. doi:10.1177/1077559516657890.

Douglas, E. M., & Hines, D. A. (2011). The helpseeking experiences of men who sustain intimate partner violence: An overlooked population and implications for practice. *Journal of Family Violence, 26*(6), 473–485.

Douglas, E. M., & Mohn, B. L. (2014). Fatal and non-fatal child maltreatment in the US: An analysis of child, caregiver, and service utilization with the National Child Abuse and Neglect Data Set. *Child Abuse & Neglect, 38*(1), 42–51. doi: http://dx.doi.org/10.1016/j.chiabu.2013.10.022.

Douglas, E. M., Mohn, B. L., & Gushwa, M. (2015). The presence of maltreatment fatality-related content in pre-service child welfare training curricula: A brief report of 20 states. *Child and Adolescent Social Work Journal, 32*(3), 213–218.

Douglas, E. M., & Serino, P. J. (2013). The extent of evidence-based information about child maltreatment fatalities in social science textbooks. *Journal of Evidence-Based Social Work, 10*(5), 447–454. doi:10.1080/15433714.2012.759839.

Durfee, M., Durfee, D. T., & West, M. P. (2002). Child fatality review: An international movement. *Child Abuse & Neglect, 26*, 619–636.

Fein, L. G. (1979). Can child fatalities, end product child abuse, be prevented? *Children and Youth Services Review, 1*, 31–53.

Finkelhor, D., & Jones, L. (2006). Why have child maltreatment and child victimization declined? *Journal of Social Issues, 62*(4), 685–716.

Finkelhor, D., & Jones, L. M. (2012). *Have sexual abuse and physical abuse declined since the 1990s?* Durham, NH: Crimes Against Children Research Center, University of New Hampshire.

Gelles, R. J. (1996). *The book of David: How preserving families can cost children's lives.* New York, NY: Basic Books.

Gibbs, D., Rojas-Smith, L., Wetterhall, S., Farris, T., Schnitzer, P. G., Leeb, R. T., et al. (2013). Improving identification of child maltreatment fatalities through public health surveillance. *Journal of Public Child Welfare, 7*(1), 1–19. doi:10.1080/15548732.2012.671032.

Herman-Giddens, M. E., Brown, G., Verbiest, S., Carlson, P. J., Hooten, E. G., Howell, E., et al. (1999). Underascertainment of child abuse mortality in the United States. *JAMA, 282*(5), 463–467.

Hewes, H. A., Keenan, H. T., McDonnell, W. M., Dudley, N. C., & Herman, B. E. (2011). Judicial outcomes of child abuse homicide. *Archives of Pediatrics and Adolescent Medicine, 165*(10), 918–921. doi:10.1001/archpediatrics.2011.151.

Hochstadt, N. J. (2006). Child death review teams: A vital component of child protection. *Child Welfare, 85*(4), 653–670.

Jason, J. (1984). Centers for Disease Control and the epidemiology of violence. *Child Abuse & Neglect, 8*(3), 279–283.

Jenny, C., & Isaac, R. (2006). The relation between child death and child maltreatment. *Archives of Disease in Childhood, 91*(3), 265–269.

Johnson, C. F. (2000). Death from child abuse and neglect. *Lancet, 356*, s14–s14.

Jones, L. M., & Finkelhor, D. (2003). Putting together evidence on declining trends in sexual abuse: A complex puzzle. *Child Abuse & Neglect, 27*(2), 133–135.

Jones, L. M., Finkelhor, D., & Halter, S. (2006). Child maltreatment trends in the 1990s: Why does neglect differ from sexual and physical abuse? *Child Abuse & Neglect, 11*(2), 107–120.

Jones, L. M., Finkelhor, D., & Kopiec, K. (2001). Why is sexual abuse declining? A survey of state child protection administrators. *Child Abuse & Neglect, 25*(9), 1139–1158.

Kemp, S. P., Marcenko, M. O., Lyons, S. J., & Kruzich, J. M. (2014). Strength-based practice and parental engagement in child welfare services: An empirical examination. *Children and Youth Services Review, 47*, 27–35. doi:10.1016/j.childyouth.2013.11.001.

Kim, S. Y., Shapiro-Mendoza, C. K., Chu, S. Y., Camperlengo, L. T., & Anderson, R. N. (2012). Differentiating cause-of-death terminology for deaths coded as sudden infant death syndrome, accidental suffocation, and unknown cause: An investigation using US death certificates, 2003–2004. *Journal of Forensic Sciences, 57*(2), 364–369. doi:10.1111/j.1556-4029.2011.01937.x.

Klevens, J., & Leeb, R. T. (2010). Child maltreatment fatalities in children under 5: Findings from the National Violence Death Reporting System. *Child Abuse & Neglect: The International Journal, 34*(4), 262–266.

Korbin, J. E. (1987). Incarcerated mothers' perceptions and interpretations of their fatally maltreated children. *Child Abuse & Neglect, 11*, 397–407.

Korbin, J. E. (1998). "Good mothers," "Babykillers" and fatal child maltreatment. In N. Scheper-Hughes & C. Sargent (Eds.), *Small wars: The cultural politics of childhood* (pp. 253–276). Berkeley, CA/Los Angeles, CA: University of California Press.

Leeb, R. T., Paulozzi, L. J., Melanson, C., Simon, T. R., & Arias, I. (2008). *Child maltreatment surveillance: Uniform definitions for public health and recommended data elements*. Atlanta, GA: Centers for Disease Control & Prevention. Retrieved from http://www.cdc.gov/violenceprevention/pdf/cm_surveillance-a.pdf

Lietz, C. A. (2011). Theoretical adherence to family centered practice: Are strengths-based principles illustrated in families' descriptions of child welfare services? *Children and Youth Services Review, 33*(6), 888–893. doi:10.1016/j.childyouth.2010.12.012.

Lietz, C. A., & Rounds, T. (2009). Strengths-based supervision: A child welfare supervision training project. *Clinical Supervisor, 28*(2), 124–140. doi:10.1080/07325220903334065.

Mapp, S. C. (2002). A framework for family visiting for children in long-term foster care. *Families in Society, 83*(2), 175–182.

Martin, J. A., Hamilton, B. E., Osterman, M. J. K., Curtin, S. C., & Matthews, T. J. (2013). Births: Final data for 2012. *National Vital Statistics Report, 62*(9). http://www.cdc.gov/nchs/data/nvsr/nvsr62/nvsr62_09.pdf

McClain, P. W., Sacks, J. J., Froehlke, R. G., & Ewigman, B. G. (1993). Estimates of fatal child abuse and neglect, United States, 1979 though 1988. *Pediatrics, 91*(2), 338–434.

Meara, E. (1999). DHS target of attacks at hearing. *Bangor Daily News*.

Mor Barak, M. Ã. l. E., Levin, A., Nissly, J. A., & Lane, C. J. (2006). Why do they leave? Modeling child welfare workers' turnover intentions. *Children and Youth Services Review, 28*(5), 548–577.

National Center for the Prosecution of Child Abuse. (2013). *Child abuse crimes: Child homicide*. Retrieved December 31, 2014, from http://www.ndaa.org/pdf/ChildHomicide 2013.pdf

National Conference of State Legislatures. (2011). Summary of the "Child and Family Services Improvement and Innovation Act" (S.1542/H.R. 2883). Retrieved December 21, 2013, from http://www.ncsl.org/research/human-services/summary-of-the-quotchild-and-family-services-imp.aspx

Oberman, M. (2008). Comment: Infant abandonment in Texas. *Child Maltreatment, 13*(1), 94–95.

Olds, D. L., Eckenrode, J., Henderson, C. R., Jr., et al. (1997). Long-term effects of home visitation on maternal life course and child abuse and neglect: Fifteen-year follow-up of a randomized trial. *JAMA, 278*(8), 637–643. doi:10.1001/jama.1997.03550080047038.

Olds, D. L., Kitzman, H., Knudtson, M. D., Anson, E., Smith, J. A., & Cole, R. (2014). Effect of home visiting by nurses on maternal and child mortality: Results of a 2-decade follow-up of a randomized clinical trial. *JAMA Pediatrics, 168*(9), 800–806. doi:10.1001/jamapediatrics.2014.472.

Ontiveros, S. (2014, February 14). Pass the word, Illinois' safe haven law works. *Chicago Sun-Times*. Retrieved from http://www.suntimes.com/news/ontiveros/25546348-452/pass-the-word-illinois-safe-haven-law-works.html-.U5oQ8vldU6w

Onwuachi-Saunders, C., Forjuoh, S. N., West, P., & Brooks, C. (1999). Child death reviews: A gold mine for injury prevention and control. *Injury Prevention, 5*(276-279).

Otis, G. A. (2014, February 9). Administration for children's services failing to prevent tragedies despite city efforts to make changes. *Daily News.* Retrieved from http://www.nydailynews.com/new-york/administration-children-services-failing-prevent-tragedies-article-1.1607516

Palusci, V. J., & Covington, T. M. (2014). Child maltreatment deaths in the U.S. National Child Death Review Case Reporting System. *Child Abuse & Neglect, 38*(1), 25–36. doi: http://dx.doi.org/10.1016/j.chiabu.2013.08.014.

Palusci, V. J., Wirtz, S. J., & Covington, T. M. (2010). Using capture-recapture methods to better ascertain the incidence of fatal child maltreatment. *Child Abuse & Neglect: The International Journal, 34*(6), 396–402.

Palusci, V. J., Yager, S., & Covington, T. M. (2010). Effects of a Citizens Review Panel in preventing child maltreatment fatalities. *Child Abuse & Neglect, 34*(5), 324–331.

Phipps, C. A. (1999). Responding to child homicide: A statutory proposal. *The Journal of Criminal Law and Criminology, 89*(2), 535–613.

Pitzl, M. J. (2014, May 16). New agency, new name: State seeks new moniker for CPS. *The Republic.* Retrieved from http://www.azcentral.com/story/news/politics/2014/05/17/new-agency-new-name-state-seeks-new-moniker-cps/9206707/

Poole, M. K., Seal, D. W., & Taylor, C. A. (2014). A systematic review of universal campaigns targeting child physical abuse prevention. *Health Education Research, 29*(3), 388–432. doi:10.1093/her/cyu012.

Prinz, R. J., Sanders, M. R., Shapiro, C. J., Whitaker, D. J., & Lutzker, J. R. (2009). Population-based prevention of child maltreatment: The U.S. triple P system population trial. *Prevention Science, 10*(1), 1–12.

Putnam-Hornstein, E., Wood, J. N., Fluke, J., Yoshioka-Maxwell, A., & Berger, R. P. (2013). Preventing severe and fatal child maltreatment: Making the case for the expanded use and integration of data. *Child Welfare, 92*(2), 59–75.

Richmond-Crum, M., Joyner, C., Fogerty, S., Ellis, M. L., & Saul, J. (2013). Applying a public health approach: The role of state health departments in preventing maltreatment and fatalities of children. *Child Welfare, 92*(2), 99–117.

Rizzi, T., & Hinko, C. (2011, January 28). Children of Hope becomes Tim Jaccard's safe haven. *Farmingdale Observer.* Retrieved from http://www.antonnews.com/farmingdaleobserver/news/13120-children-of-hope-becomes-tim-jaccards-safe-haven.html

Roose, R., Roets, G., & Schiettecat, T. (2014). Implementing a strengths perspective in child welfare and protection: A challenge not to be taken lightly. *European Journal of Social Work, 17*(1), 3–17. doi:10.1080/13691457.2012.739555.

Schnitzer, P. G., Gulino, S. P., & Ying-Ying, T. Y. (2013). Advancing public health surveillance to estimate child maltreatment fatalities: Review and recommendations. *Child Welfare, 92*(2), 77–98.

Shapiro-Mendoza, C. K., Kimball, M., Tomashek, K. M., Anderson, R. N., & Blanding, S. (2009). US infant mortality trends attributable to accidental suffocation and strangulation in bed from 1984 through 2004: Are rates increasing? *Pediatrics, 123*(2), 533–539. doi:10.1542/peds.2007-3746.

Staudt, M., Howard, M. O., & Drake, B. (2001). The operationalization, implementation, and effectiveness of the strengths perspective: A review of empirical studies. *Journal of Social Service Research, 27*(3), 1–21.

Straus, M. A., Douglas, E. M., & Medeiros, R. A. (2014). *The primordial violence: Corporal punishment by parents, cognitive development, and crime.* New York, NY: Routledge.

Tilkin, D. (2013, November 7). Fallen followers: Investigation finds 10 mire dead children of faith healers. *KATU-TV.* Retrieved from http://www.katu.com/news/investigators/Fallen-followers-Investigation-finds-10-more-dead-children-of-faith-healers-231050911.html

Travis, D. J., & Mor Barak, M. Ã. l. E. (2010). Fight or flight? Factors influencing child welfare workers' propensity to seek positive change or disengage from their jobs. *Journal of Social Service Research, 36*(3), 188–205.

U.S. Commission to End Child Abuse and Neglect Fatalities. (2016). *Within our reach: A national strategy to eliminate child abuse and neglect fatalities*. Retrieved from http://www.acf.hhs.gov/programs/cb/resource/cecanf-final-report.

U.S. Department of Health & Human Services. (2015). *Child maltreatment 2012: Reports from the States to the National Child Abuse and Neglect Data Systems – National statistics on child abuse and neglect*. Washington, DC: Administration for Children & Families, U.S. Department of Health & Human Services.

United States Advisory Board on Child Abuse and Neglect. (1995). *A nation's shame: Fatal child abuse and neglect in the United States*.

Vincent, S. (2010). *Preventing child deaths: Learning from review*. Edinburgh, UK: Dunedin Academic Press Ltd.

Webster, R. A., Schnitzer, P. G., Jenny, C., Ewigman, B. G., & Alario, A. J. (2003). Child death review: The state of the nation. *American Journal of Prevention Medicine, 25*(5), 58–64.

Wirtz, S. J., Foster, V., & Lenart, G. A. (2011). Assessing and improving child death review team recommendations. *Injury Prevention, 17*, 64–70.

Yampolskaya, S., Greenbaum, P. E., & Berson, I. R. (2009). Profiles of child maltreatment perpetrators and risk for fatal assault: A latent class analysis. *Journal of Family Violence, 24*(5), 337–348.

Index

A
Abandoned/discarded infants
    Abandoned Infants Assistance Act, 95
    child welfare services, 92
    definition, 91, 92
    foundling hospitals, 94
Abusive head trauma (AHT). *See* Shaken baby syndrome (SBS)

C
Child death review, 71–86
    child death review teams, 72–74
        composition of, 72–74, 84
        funding of, 72, 80, 84
        origins of, 71
        outputs, 71, 75–77
        purpose/focus of
            prevention, 72–74
            prosecution, 72, 73
        recommendations from, 75–78, 83, 85, 86
        state policy, 73, 78, 86
    child welfare internal review, 74, 79
    Child Welfare League of America, 55, 79
    criticism, 80, 81, 83
    effectiveness of, 71, 77, 84, 154
    international approaches
        Child death overview panels, 81, 82
        Public inquiry, 81, 82
    National Center for the Review and Prevention of Child Deaths, 72, 74, 75, 80, 84, 85, 119
    National Center on Child Fatality Review (*see* Child death review, National Center for the Review and Prevention of Child Deaths)
    National Child Death Review Case Reporting System, 28–30, 32, 34, 80, 83, 84
Child maltreatment, 11, 13, 80, 127, 128, 132, 134, 135, 137–142, 150, 151, 153, 158, 159, 161
    abuse, 9–11, 20, 22, 35–39, 110, 112, 116, 119, 121, 130
    data sources
        National Child Abuse and Neglect Data, 150, 151, 158
        National Data Archive on Child Abuse and Neglect, 80, 151
    death (*see* Child maltreatment fatality)
    neglect, medical, 12, 15–16, 116, 122
    neglect, physical, 12, 15, 55, 91
    neglect, supervisory
        motor vehicles, inside of, 11, 14, 127, 134, 141, 158
        safe sleep, co-sleeping, 135, 158
        water, around, 13, 14, 132, 134, 141, 153
    prevention of
        home-visiting programs, 128, 137, 138, 141, 142
        parenting education, 138–140, 142, 159, 161
Child maltreatment fatality, 3, 5, 6, 9–12, 19–22, 28–30, 32, 34, 36, 40, 50, 52, 79, 80, 83, 84, 113, 114, 122, 150–152, 158
    causes of death, 13, 14, 18, 19, 52, 72, 141, 153, 159

Child maltreatment fatality (*cont.*)
  data sources
    Centers for Disease Control and Prevention, 6, 19, 28, 50, 79, 113
    Federal Bureau of Investigation, 19
    National Child Abuse and Neglect Data Set, 11, 12, 20, 30, 32, 36, 40, 84, 150–152, 158
    National Child Death Review Case Reporting System, 28–30, 32, 34, 80, 83, 84
  definition
    child homicide, 10, 114
    filicide, 10
    infanticide, 10
    neonaticide, 10
  Europe, 18, 94, 118
  fatality lens, 157, 161
  interest in, 82
  medical examiner, 9, 18, 19, 21, 22, 35, 39, 73, 74, 94, 103, 110–112, 158
  prevalence rate trends, changes in, 6, 9, 21, 22, 52, 122
  prevention of, 71
  recommendations for change, 81, 82, 128, 149, 155
  research, lack of, 16
  risk factors
    child, 6
    household, 6
    mental health, 3
    parent, 6
    parent-child relationship, 6
    violence or domestic violence, 5
Child welfare profession/professionals, 61–63
  assessing for risk factors for fatality, 48, 65
  beliefs and concerns about fatalities, 49
  child maltreatment fatality and consequences of (*see* Child maltreatment fatality)
  child welfare practice before fatality, 48–49, 55–59, 65
  child welfare services before fatality, 54, 56, 59
  knowledge of risk factors for fatality, 48, 50–51, 53, 56
  post-traumatic stress
    after fatality, 61
    beliefs about fatality, 62
    support for workers after fatality, 62–63
  strength-based approach, 57
  training in risk factors for fatality, 48, 51–53, 55
  who experience death of child client, 53–59
Children's Healthcare Is a Legal Duty (CHILD), 116, 118, 155, 159
Co-sleeping. *See* Child maltreatment, neglect—supervisory
Criminal justice responses, 114–116, 118–121
  barriers to prosecution, 85
  child death investigations, 110
  child death laws, 110
  Children's Healthcare Is a Legal Duty, 116, 118, 155, 159
  co-sleeping, 110
  increased penalties
    efficacy, 114–116, 118–121
  prosecution, 111, 112, 114, 116
  public perception, 65
  religions exemptions to child maltreatment, 122
  religious shield laws and child maltreatment, 116

F
Federal government
  Department of Health and Human Services, 12, 94
  U.S. Commission to Eliminate Child Abuse & Neglect Fatalities, 57, 65

M
Motor vehicles. *See* Child maltreatment, neglect—supervisory

N
National Child Abuse and Neglect Data System (NCANDS), 11, 12, 20, 30, 32, 36, 40, 84, 150–152, 158

P
Perpetrators
  fathers, 31
  mothers, 31, 32, 42, 50, 149
  parents' partner, 31
Prevention, child maltreatment. *See* Child maltreatment, prevention of
Prevention, public health levels of, 6, 127, 149, 160

S

Safe haven laws. *See also* Abandoned/
    discarded infants
  adoption, 91, 96, 101, 104, 105
  crime control theater, 101
  effectiveness of, 91, 105
  history, 94–99
  infant abandonments and prosecution,
    92–99, 101, 105
  National Safe Haven Alliance, 96
  non-relinquishing parents
    legal rights, 104
    notification, 105
  public education/marketing of, 91, 92, 101,
    103–104, 106
  safe haven locations, 91, 98–102,
    104, 105
  safe haven receivers, 100

Save Abandoned Babies Foundation,
    Illinois, 100–103, 106
  state policies, 99, 101
  use of, 91
Safe sleep. *See* Child
    maltreatment, neglect—supervisory
Shaken baby syndrome (SBS), 131, 140
  New York, 130
  prevention
    PURPLE program, 131, 140
  state policy, 74, 75
State policy, 73, 78, 86, 99
Strength-based approach in social work, 57, 158

U

U.S. Commission to End Child Abuse and
    Neglect Fatalities, 141, 150, 155

The manufacturer's authorised representative in the EU is Springer Nature Customer Service Centre GmbH, Europaplatz 3, 69115 Heidelberg, Germany. If you have any concerns regarding our products, please contact ProductSafety@springernature.com

Printed and bound by CPI Group (UK) Ltd, Croydon, CR0 4YY

26/03/2026

02078915-0002